DEATH BY PRESCRIPTION

DEATH BY PRESCRIPTION

A FATHER TAKES ON HIS DAUGHTER'S
KILLER—THE MULTI-BILLION-DOLLAR
PHARMACEUTICAL INDUSTRY

Terence H. Young

KEY PORTER BOOKS

Library and Archives Canada Cataloguing in Publication

Young, Terence
    Death by prescription : a father takes on his daughter's killer— the multi-billion dollar pharmaceutical industry / Terence Young.

ISBN 978-1-55263-825-5

    1. Young, Vanessa—Death and burial. 2. Drugs—Side effects. 3. Cisapride. 4. Pharmaceutical industry. 5. Pharmaceutical policy— Canada. I. Title.

HD9670.C32Y69 2009   338.4'761510971   C2006-906436-9

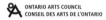

The publisher gratefully acknowledges the support of the Canada Council for the Arts and the Ontario Arts Council for its publishing program. We acknowledge the support of the Government of Ontario through the Ontario Media Development Corporation's Ontario Book Initiative.

We acknowledge the financial support of the Government of Canada through the Book Publishing Industry Development Program (BPIDP) for our publishing activities.

Key Porter Books Limited
Six Adelaide Street East, Tenth Floor
Toronto, Ontario
Canada M5C 1H6

www.keyporter.com

Text design: Marijke Friesen
Electronic formatting: Alison Carr

Printed and bound in Canada

09 10 11 12 13 5 4 3 2 1

Vanessa Charlotte Young

A RARE AND BRILLIANT LIGHT
LOVING, CARING, FORGIVING
HOME WITH THE ANGELS
AND FOREVER IN OUR HEARTS

These words appear on Vanessa's grave marker
at Mount Pleasant Cemetery in Toronto.

This book is dedicated to Vanessa.
Born April 8, 1984
Died March 19, 2000

It is also dedicated to Gloria, Madeline, and Hart.

CONTENTS

IN THIS BOOK ALL OF THE PEOPLE ARE REAL. Some of the names have been changed to avoid litigation for them and me, and so that those who confided in me don't lose their jobs and careers. Otherwise I could simply not tell this story.

Conversations with various parties were recreated here to the best of my ability from memory, using notes I made during interviews and telephone calls, from personal emails, and occasionally sourced in more than one communication.

From all the wonderful stories, the books, poems and songs throughout history we are conditioned to believe that the highest form of love is romantic love between a man and a woman. But the unconditional love connecting the vulnerability of a child with the protection of a loving parent transcends this world in a special way. Nothing could be more important to our humanity. It is the most common way that ordinary people get a chance to be like a loving Creator. Anyone that intentionally undermines that protection is committing an undeniable wrong. No society should tolerate it for any reason.

Warning

Do not stop taking your prescriptions based on anything you read in this book, which could be dangerous. Stopping a prescription or changing a prescription should only be done with the advice of a qualified and well-informed doctor who is familiar with your medical history, your condition, with all other drugs you are taking, and with the foods and liquids you are consuming.

New Years Day, 1997
Women's College Hospital, Toronto—Neonatal
Intensive Care Unit

Adelaide Morrison weighed 2 lbs 8 oz when she was born.

She had a problem spitting up but was being given the motility drug Prepulsid (cisapride) in her feeding tube to help her digest food, and was gaining weight. After a month in the NICU she was moved to a step-down unit for stronger "preemies." Her mother, Sarah—a nurse—was hopeful she could take her home soon.

Then an alarm: Adelaide began to develop bradycardia—slow heartbeat. Adelaide was taken back into the NICU on New Year's Eve. Her tiny heart slowed to half the normal rate. No one could explain why this was happening. Filled with dread, her parents were afraid this was the end.

Then, just as the NICU nurse was putting the cisapride into her feeding tube her doctor burst into the NICU crying out, "Take it out. Take it out. No more cisapride." She stopped.

The doctor had just read a study in a medical journal about an infant who had died after being given cisapride. Adelaide was rushed to nearby Sick Children's Hospital and her parents waited and prayed through the night as the rhythm in her tiny heart returned to normal. Today Adelaide is a happy, healthy eleven-year-old who studies dance and voice.

July 1999—Orangeville, Ontario

A twenty-one-year-old woman had experienced repeated terrifying episodes.

"I'd walk across the room and think I was going to die, like my heart was jumping out of my chest."[1] *Sometimes she had to grab a table to keep from passing out. Her family doctor and specialist told her she was just anxious. Neither mentioned the Prepulsid she was taking or told her she should stop it. Instinctively she decided to stop taking Prepulsid on her own and the episodes ended.*

Other people who took Prepulsid weren't as lucky. This is one story of many.

SECTION ONE

No One is Safe

Chapter 1

A Night of Terror

March 19, 2000

GLORIA AND I HAD BEEN OUT SHOPPING. It was a typical cloudy Saturday afternoon in March. Our fifteen-year-old daughter, Vanessa, was somewhat of a homebody, and that Saturday she stayed home to listen to music, talk on the phone, and bake cookies. We had just renewed her prescription for Prepulsid earlier in the afternoon. Her problem of throwing up after meals was under control, but she felt the pills helped her, and had been taking them that week when she felt bloated. Her symptoms didn't occur all the time but on and off, perhaps related to stress or social pressure we were told. Our family doctor had directed Vanessa to take Prepulsid as needed to help move food through her system. We took the problem quite seriously like any good parents and watched her closely. Our doctor had never mentioned any safety concerns with Prepulsid. We viewed it like a kind of super Rolaids. Like any popular teenager on a Saturday evening, she was making plans to go out, something that normally required some negotiations with her mother and me.

Our other daughter, Madeline, aged seventeen, was out with friends. Our son, Hart, aged thirteen, was in his room. That afternoon Vanessa had called to say she was baking cookies and asked when we'd be home. Of course she said "I love you Dad." Sometimes that was her sole purpose for calling. We arrived home after six, a little tired and ready for dinner.

I sat down in the front room, my study, to read the weekend paper and Gloria went upstairs. Vanessa came down to greet me.

Everything from that moment on is a kind of slow-motion blur to me, more like a gripping nightmare that won't go away than reality. It has been replayed over and over in my mind, like we were all in a horror movie. She wanted to ask me something. I remember saying to her, "Not now, Vanessa," so I could consider the inevitable request to discuss her curfew until after dinner when I was refreshed and in a better frame of mind.

I see it all now in slow motion: she jumped up to head back upstairs and in midair fell back, hitting the back of her head on the carpeted floor with a thump, as if she had been pushed by a giant invisible hand.

Immediately I rushed to her, thinking perhaps it was a joke that went wrong, asking her if she was okay. She was limp, silent, motionless, and pale.

A feeling deep inside me told me something was terribly wrong. This was not just a fainting spell, and Vanessa had never fainted before. The first aid training I'd had years before kicked in and I put my index finger to her carotid artery. I could feel no pulse, no beat, nothing.

"God, what is happening?"

Maybe I was too nervous and just couldn't find a pulse. Maybe my fingers were in the wrong place. Maybe I forgot exactly where to check. No, they were in the right place. I *knew* I should remain in control, but I was being overwhelmed by horror. *What was happening?*

"Gloria!" I shouted upstairs. No answer.

"Hart! Call Uncle Ted!"

Gloria came running down the stairs following Hart, terrified by my tone. Hart had a frozen, confused look of fear on his face, I guess because I had shouted the telephone number at him. I still feel a terrible ache when I remember what I was forced to put him through. He was only thirteen years old. I fumbled for my cellphone and dialed the number.

Uncle Ted is my oldest brother, Dr. J.E.M. Young, a surgeon in Hamilton, Ontario, a half-hour away. I was so thankful. He was on the phone immediately. Thank God, I breathed in relief. I tried as calmly as I could to tell him what had happened. I could hear my own voice as if I was in a dream. Ted was calm, professional. "If there is no pulse, call an ambulance. Give her mouth-to-mouth resuscitation."

I shouted again at Hart to go over and get our neighbour two doors down—Anna—a nurse. I prayed she was home. Perhaps thirty seconds had gone by. How long can someone live without breathing? Ridiculously, I remembered a number of eight minutes from a book I'd read in high school. A human brain can live eight minutes without oxygen before it starts to die. But I also knew the brain can live longer if it gets oxygen. Gloria had called an ambulance. The paramedics were on the way. The phone was ringing. Commotion. I had begun giving Vanessa mouth-to-mouth resuscitation before Hart was out the door.

From that moment on I focused on trying to pour the life back into Vanessa, and prayed.

I blew into her mouth while holding her nose, and turned my head to listen for the air to come out, hoping she would start breathing on her own. Her chest rose with each breath. But she was not breathing on her own. *Come on Vanessa. Come on sweetheart. You can do it. You can't leave us. Breathe in. Breathe! This can't be happening. God, where are you?*

The phone was still ringing.

Anna burst into the room and within seconds was on my cellular phone with Ted. Then she was beside me. She checked for a pulse and asked me to stop. She attempted to revive Vanessa with CPR—pushing on her chest to try and start her heart. It wasn't working. Anna is calm but I can tell she is frustrated. How long has it been? I wonder. Anna stops the CPR. I start mouth-to-mouth again.

I screamed in my mind, "God where are you? Please don't let his happen!" Scenarios played through my mind like a movie. Vanessa would start to breathe and sit up and hug me. The paramedics would get her heart going. She would be fine. Tomorrow we'd laugh about this. Then, a reversal. She would die on our floor.

Our lives would never be the same.

No. Nothing had changed. I continued blowing into her mouth and holding her nose, then letting the air escape. *Where are the paramedics? Why is this happening?* Anna tries CPR again.

Then they arrived. Some relief. It had not been over eight minutes. She could still be fine. They asked me and Anna to step into the other room. A police officer was standing in front of me. I'm not sure exactly when he'd arrived.

"Was she on any medication?"

"Huh? Uh, yes, she takes Prepulsid to help her with bloating."

"Is she taking anything else?"

"No."

"Are you sure?"

"Yes, absolutely."

"Could she have taken any recreational drugs?"

"No. She would never do that."

"Could she have taken any other medication?"

"No! We are very careful with drugs. She was fine today.

She was baking cookies. She probably ate some of them. Nothing like this has ever happened before. There is no reason for this to happen."

I don't remember who asked the questions, but I think it was one of the paramedics—the one talking into the two-way radio.

"Can you check her room and belongings?" Gloria and I ran upstairs and tore through Vanessa's purse, bathroom drawer, bedclothes, pants pockets, and drawers—every private place she had and dumped it all on the bed. Nothing. No Tylenol. No aspirin. No anything whatsoever. No pills other than her prescription for Prepulsid.

We ran downstairs. The paramedics had cut Vanessa's sweatshirt up the middle to expose her chest and stomach. I quietly prayed for the day we could take her out and buy a new one. Vanessa's sister Madeline had arrived home, terrified to see the emergency vehicles in front of our house and entered the open front door and nightmarish scene. We did our best to explain.

More commotion—now slowly, imperceptibly, turning to controlled terror. Hart was standing outside the front door totally alone watching his world come down around him. Madeline and Gloria were terrified. Someone told me I should help Hart. Of course. I called him and sat beside him waiting while the emergency crews went through their life-saving routines. Nothing. I did my best to say reassuring things to Hart and Madeline but I know the terror was visible in my eyes.

The paramedics were talking on the two-way radio with the local hospital emergency staff. They had put an oxygen mask over Vanessa's face and given her a shot, and had used the paddles to shock her heart into starting to pump again. *What time was it?* I'd lost count. But I think it's a lot more than eight minutes. Maybe I was wrong. Maybe eight minutes doesn't mean anything. This is a nightmare. Please help me wake up.

They could not get Vanessa's heart going. She was on the portable gurney and out the door. Someone drove us to the hospital behind the ambulance. I don't remember who. The siren and flashing lights reminded me I was in a nightmare. We were the parents in the ambulance. We were the family going to the hospital in fear. It was my little girl whose heart had stopped. I was the guy who people looked at curiously from the sidewalk as they walked their dogs. And I had no idea why. The doctors were waiting. What was happening?

"Does Vanessa have a prolonged QT?"

"What?"

A familiar face. It was the gastroenterologist who had been one of Vanessa's doctors. She had had an appointment with Vanessa two months before. No, I answered, Vanessa had no health problems other than throwing up sometimes after meals.

I said we'd never heard of long QT. She was was sitting behind a counter at the nurses station leaning over, reading the small print in a thick blue book. I stood on the other side.

I found out later the book was the *Compendium of Pharmaceuticals and Specialties* (CPS)—the same book found in every doctor's office and pharmacy in Canada, their key drug manual. In the U.S. the equivalent manual is called *The Physician's Desk Reference* (PDR). Every doctor and pharmacist has one.

"Does she have low potassium?"

"No."

"Does she have an electrolyte disorder?"

"What is that?"

I did my best to maintain my composure and to answer her questions. But I had no idea what she was talking about.

As we spoke Vanessa had been rushed to the emergency treatment room on the gurney. She was surrounded by medical staff as they tried urgently to get her heart going again. She laid there, her chest uncovered, helpless, and innocent. Gloria,

Madeline, and Hart were in the waiting room. My brother Ted arrived from Hamilton and was observing from the door. My brother Denton and his wife Suzanne had arrived from Mississauga. There were a few faint smiles—the source of which was the faith that had sustained our family all our lives.

This would be OK. Things always were for our family.

Vanessa would recover.

I went back to where the hospital staff was trying to start Vanessa's heart and held her hand. I felt like I was floating. Our life with Vanessa flashed through my mind like a high-speed slide show.

THERE IS NOTHING MUCH that makes our family very different from any other, except perhaps our many blessings. We live in the beautiful community of Oakville, Ontario, with good schools and a low crime rate, a place Gloria and I had chosen in 1985 when we moved from Toronto. Our children had lots of things to do and many friends.

By 2000 they were getting older and were more independent. Gloria worked in public affairs for a hospital. I was a former Member of Ontario's Provincial Parliament building up my own consultancy business. My riding of Halton Centre was eliminated due to downsizing of the Ontario provincial ridings the year before. Vanessa had been a member of the Burl-Oak Canoe Club for three years and had a large circle of friends at school.

She had grown in recent years to 5'10" and 139 lbs. of graceful beauty—not just her looks, but her entire persona. Her inner beauty shone through. I could hear her soft voice and feel her thick blonde hair in my hands as she hugged me. She was very sweet and empathetic, although she had no time for "phonies." She was very aware of the rest of us at home—our ups and downs—and would easily calm any of us who'd had a bad day with a kind word. I remembered one day years before when she was ten. I sat at the kitchen table stressed out after a long day of work and one-hour commute from Toronto. She put her little hands on my back and rubbed it to calm me down. My stress melted away. That's the kind of thoughtful person she was—mature beyond her years—that brought out the best in me and others.

The Christmas before, she and her friend Jen had called up a local senior's residence to see if there were any residents who were lonely and would like to have visitors. They visited an elderly lady who wanted someone to talk to. She laughed as she told us about it. She babysat regularly for our longtime neighbours, David and Ann. They had a one-year-old girl she loved to cuddle and called "my baby." When she was younger, if she saw an elderly person walking along the street alone as we drove by she would tell me that made her feel sad. I explained that person might not be lonely at all, but just going out to buy food to make dinner for guests or family. And that some people liked to be alone. I don't think she ever really believed me. She was wise beyond her years.

The thing she did that I loved the most was leaving thoughtful notes for me at my desk when I came in late. They always said "I love you Dad." She also left kind notes for others. She would call my cellular phone any time of day just to say, "Hi Dad, see you when you get home." and never said goodbye without saying "I love you." One Friday evening, just weeks before, she told her friends that she was busy and went over to spend time with my widowed mother. For a popular fifteen-year-old to choose a visit with grandmother over her friends on Friday night is pretty special.

I couldn't imagine our life without her.

Laying there on the table, Vanessa looked so vulnerable, so beautiful yet so far away. Her heart had been stopped for a very long time. I was facing the unthinkable. We were looking for a miracle now, I thought. Was there anything I could do to help? I made one last desperate effort to try—the only thing I could do. I remembered the stories I'd heard of the near-dead coming back to life—people who described a bright light and a tunnel leading to it. I had to keep my faith that everything could still be alright. I had to try to call Vanessa back from the light. *Not yet Vanessa. It's not right. This is a mistake. Come back.*

I took her limp hand and spoke those words to her out loud, above the din of the machines and the doctors and nurses trying to start her heart, as her father—with gentle encouragement—as if it was just the two of us in the room. As if it was just the two of us in the universe. Like when she was little and had a bad dream.

"It's OK, Vanessa. You can do it. You come back now. We love you sweetheart. We are here for you. It's OK. Your Mom is waiting with Madeline and Hart. You come back to us now."

Something happened. The sound on the monitor changed. The eyes of the doctors and nurses over their sanitary breathing masks darted from side to side. Nobody said anything. Then the doctor in charge told me to keep speaking to her. I did. The sound changed again.

A heartbeat! The monitor began to bleep. Her heart had started again. Her face and body flushed with healthy colour. I could tell from the eyes over the masks around me that this was surprising, unexpected. She seemed stabilized. The nightmare wasn't over, but her heart was pumping at least. At least they had started her heart.

One step at a time.

I hurried to the waiting room to tell my family they had started Vanessa's heart. Then I went back out to our doctor. I had a lot of questions. She was the on-duty specialist that evening and still sat at the nurse's station.

I asked her what a long QT was and what Prepulsid had to do with Vanessa's collapse. I referred to the motility test.

"What do you mean?" she asked. "Is Vanessa one of my patients?"

I had assumed she remembered that Vanessa had been taking Prepulsid periodically. Back in January she had recommended a motility test at McMaster University Medical Centre to see if Vanessa had any blockage in her system that caused throwing up.

"Yes she was." I reminded her about the motility test.

"Did I prescribe Prepulsid for her?"

Just then a nurse called me to the phone at the nurse's station. It was Dr. Kayner on the line from the hospital where he was on duty. Perhaps someone had alerted him. He had cared for Vanessa since she was two years old. He asked me about what had happened. I assumed he had been briefed on the phone by the emergency staff. Vanessa's heart had been stopped for a long time, but was at least pumping again.

"Bring her into the office on Monday to see me," he said.

I was shocked: He had no idea what was going on. No one had told him one of his patients had been technically dead for almost half an hour!

"This sounds like Seldane all over again," he said.

I had no idea what that meant. I mumbled something, trying to sound positive, literally afraid to say out loud that it may be too late. I thanked him and hung up, praying that Vanessa would actually be able to visit anyone on Monday, and that it was me who was out of touch with reality, not him.

My brother Ted had been monitoring Vanessa's care and told me that she was being sent to intensive care. The heart specialist who had revived her heart, Dr. Eggar, was on his way home, exhausted. Vanessa would need a neurologist now. I stopped him to thank him and asked, "What's this about Prepulsid?"

He shook his head. "They dish it out like water."

God, I thought. Don't tell me this was all caused by some careless error. I asked him a few more questions but my mind had blanked out. I couldn't absorb anything else.

My brother Ted advised us to move her to McMaster University Medical Centre for specialist care. We agreed. Ted drove me following the ambulance. Someone drove Gloria home where she stopped to pick up some things. The phone rang, she told me later. It was Dr. Kayner. Gloria said he asked if he had prescribed Prepulsid for Vanessa. Gloria told him he had, just before she rushed out the door.

Ted and his wife Linda were at the hospital with us all night, and offered their nearby home for respite. My brother Scot and his wife Amanda joined us in our vigil into the next day. Ted called in a specialist he knew to come in and try to help. He and his colleagues at McMaster tried valiantly to help Vanessa. Some time the next morning I called our minister, Archdeacon Alex Hewitt, to ask him to pray for Vanessa at church services that morning. He promised to do so. I hadn't lost faith yet, but Vanessa's condition was deteriorating. She lay in an intensive care bed in silence, stabilized but with no sign of regaining consciousness.

Sometime in the middle of the night I laid down exhausted on a couch in the intensive care waiting room. I think it was then that it crept up on me. I don't know the exact moment. Perhaps it was when I was half-asleep. I guess the time that had passed with her heart stopped and the looks on the doctors faces, their choice of words . . . it all added up. There would be no miracle for Vanessa. I felt so guilty and ashamed that I had lost hope. I felt that I had betrayed her.

Vanessa died the next day.

We were driven home, all of us in a sickening trance, lost in our own grief.

My memory of those next days is sketchy, like trying to

tune in a distant radio station. Sometimes it's clear and you can hear every word, and others it's just noise. Of the things I remember clearly the most horrible was going to the funeral home and choosing a casket for our little girl. It was painful enough when I had to do that for my father who had died at age seventy-six, eight years before. But for Vanessa it was a cruel nightmare.

"This looks like a beauty. What kind of wood is that? How much is it? We'll take that one." All I wanted to do was run away. I wanted to turn the clock back. I wanted to wake up from the nightmare. I wanted to be off this earth and with Vanessa— to hold her in my arms again. I felt like I was in a different world. I had to step outside myself in the coming weeks and months. Nothing has ever been the same—and never will be. Everything seems surreal to this very day.

Why did this happen?

I had to find the answer. So I set out on a journey. I began the day after Vanessa died.

Chapter 2

"They Dish it Out Like Water"

"The power to do good is also the power to do harm."
—Milton Friedman

Monday, March 20, 2000
Day one of our new life

OF COURSE I HAD NO CHOICE. To do any less than find out why Vanessa died would be unthinkable. The emergency staff who had tried to revive Vanessa had asked about Prepulsid. Why? "They dish it out like water," Dr. Eggar had said. Who were "they"? Did *they* know about risks or side effects? Where would I start?

Every waking moment was surreal. I prayed that I would wake up and discover it was all a horrible dream. Of course it was very real. People were going to work as they always did. Spring break was over. The children in Oakville were heading back to school that sunny Monday morning, the girls shouting cheerfully and skipping past our front window. Everything else was the same as it always was.

We would never be the same.

Vanessa had been stolen from us, as if she was snatched off the street. She had no chance to say goodbye. She was alone in the cold morgue at McMaster University Medical Centre. I purposely blocked out a lot of things in those days, like the unthinkable things that would happen to her body there. We had been warned the hospital must do an autopsy. I thanked God for the faith my parents had instilled in me. Vanessa's spirit was in a better place. You can't hurt a spirit.

I did my best to be strong for Gloria, Madeline, and Hart. You try to smile a little. You chat about what happens next in a very mature controlled way. You bottle up your emotions. But whoever coined the phrase "broken heart" had it right. I actually felt like my heart was breaking; not just emotional pain, but real physical pain. But watching my family's pain was the hardest part. We were all acting. Going through the motions. The grief multiplies. Like an evil blooming thing.

There was a place inside each of us that had been Vanessa. It was now a hollowed-out space, empty. But it was more than that. I had always believed that the world was a good place, because the vast majority of people do the right thing. And we taught our children that same belief. Neither Gloria's family nor mine had ever suffered a tragedy. We had been truly blessed. We had every reason to get up every morning and face each day with joy and optimism.

Today was very different. Today was the first day that we faced our world with a deep . . . and unappeasable sadness. Yes. Vanessa was gone. But there was *no reason why*. Our loss felt quite meaningless to us.

I am not unworldly. I'd been in business for twenty-five years, and had been a member of provincial parliament for four years. I knew that people make mistakes. I knew they try to cover them up. But this was simply unbelievable. We have no hereditary disease of any kind on either side of the family. We had done so much to protect our children. I was the father that put the little plastic safety plugs in the electrical sockets when our children were learning to crawl and then the soft protectors on the corners of cabinets at head level when they learned to walk. We had been very careful with their health. And we had always been very cautious with prescription drugs. Our children were only allowed to take one Tylenol or ibuprofen for a headache or low-grade fever—*after* asking our permission. My God, we wouldn't even allow laxatives in the house.

We were fully aware of Vanessa starting on Prepulsid. No one had cautioned us in any way. If they had, we wouldn't have let her take it, full stop. There was simply no reason I could imagine why Vanessa should have fallen down dead. It wasn't just the bleak sadness of Vanessa's death that haunted me. The truth is I had come face to face with a startling truth: even when you try your utmost to protect the ones you love, unseen things can put them in danger. The optimism I had enjoyed for as long as I had known had been supplanted with fear.

That Monday morning I slumped over my desk, head in my hands, playing back the previous two day's events—like rewinding a movie. Tears came without control.

AT FIRST THE EMERGENCY ROOM doctors had been puzzled by Vanessa's collapse. Until they consulted a thick blue drug manual behind the counter in the Emergency Department—the *CPS*.[1] Then each one wanted to know if they were the ones that prescribed Prepulsid. Their attitude had quickly changed from puzzlement to concern about who had prescribed it.

Vanessa had followed exactly what her doctors had directed her to do. Either Gloria or I had gone with Vanessa to all her medical appointments.

From my conversations with doctors *after* they had checked the *CPS* I verified that Prepulsid was considered to be a dangerous drug for some patients—something to do with "long QT." And Dr. Kayner's statement on the phone the night Vanessa collapsed disturbed me: "This sounds like Seldane all over again." Seldane, I learned, is an antihistamine used for stuffy noses, and had been pulled off the market in 1998 for killing patients. Clearly, no one was telling me the whole story.

The first thing I had to do was warn others. I hadn't seen any sign that the doctors felt any urgency to issue a public warning, and wasn't about to wait for them to report back to us. That could take weeks. Might someone else die in the meanwhile? The very next day—before visiting the funeral home to arrange Vanessa's funeral—I got on the phone and called Johnson & Johnson's Canadian drug division, Janssen-Ortho in Toronto, the people that sold Prepulsid in Canada.

First, I wanted to tell them what had happened so they could issue an urgent public warning to patients right away to stop taking Prepulsid. A quick visit to the Johnson & Johnson website showed me that Prepulsid was sold worldwide in 119 countries. However an Internet search produced articles from U.S. news sources claiming that 341 adverse reactions had been reported in relation to "the heartburn drug Prepulsid" as well as *eighty deaths*.

This stunned me. Eighty families had gone through the grief and loss like us. All over heartburn and bloating!

Second, I wanted to ask the people at Johnson & Johnson how on earth this could happen. After leaving an urgent message, a Dr. Barton at Janssen-Ortho called me back. From that moment on I took notes during every conversation I had with anyone about Prepulsid.

"Every drug has some risk," he explained calmly. "Prepulsid has had an issue with cardiac irregularities only in the last few years." In this conversation and another one a few weeks later he told me the people at Janssen-Ortho had "been wrestling with this problem for some time," and that Health Canada wanted to restrict the drug and educate doctors. Discussion about the drug with Health Canada officials had been "on a front burner for the last few weeks." I listened in bewildered silence, desperately trying to piece together what he was saying.

There were times in the previous two days when I simply hadn't understood what the doctors were talking about. All they had to do is use one medical term I didn't know and I could be lost. Consumed with guilt, I couldn't help fearing that some time over the previous year I had not understood one of these terms. Had I missed a clue that might have saved Vanessa's life?

I am not a scientist but I certainly knew what cardiac referred to—the heart. An irregular heart was obviously bad. So this Johnson & Johnson doctor was admitting to me that Prepulsid adversely affected the hearts of some patients? That wasn't like buying irregular clothes at half price, where one sleeve was a half-inch longer than the other. An *irregular heart* could obviously be deadly. How could a drug that was made for the stomach affect the heart anyway? I thought drugs were developed to address a particular disease or part of the body.

And Janssen had been dealing with this problem for some time—the last few years. It had only been on the front burner for a few weeks? It dawned on me that I wasn't telling the people at Johnson & Johnson anything they didn't already know. Dr. Barton continued: "Four 'Dear Doctor' letters have been faxed out to the doctors. There were two warnings in the *Canadian Medical Association Journal*. It has been inappropriately pre-scribed in other cases." This was an alert of a different kind. The blame game was on. I sat forward on my chair, quickly scribbling down his words. Johnson & Johnson—the people that had made Vanessa's baby powder—had just revealed their first line of defense: It wasn't Johnson & Johnson's fault Vanessa had died. He didn't say it, but I guessed it was going to be

Dr. Kayner's fault. Because either he didn't see or didn't appreciate the significance of four "Dear Doctor" letters published for him to see. But Vanessa has seen *three other doctors* in the previous fourteen months.

Our gastroenterologist had seen Vanessa in January to test for any blockage in Vanessa's digestive system that might make her bloated and throw up after meals. The results came back negative. A little over a year before Vanessa had gone to see a psychiatrist for advice on how to deal with her bloated feeling and off-and-on problem of throwing up after meals. The doctor had diagnosed it as a mild form of bulimia. And in the previous few weeks Vanessa had seen a specialist in child psychology twice to talk about it.

Presumably these four doctors had been sent form letters from Prepulsid's manufacturer clearly outlining any dangers.

Neither Gloria nor I had ever been told, however, of any potential risks.

The language used is what I call medical-speak: words that sound less offensive than the word that describes something best. For the people at Johnson & Johnson, saying Prepulsid might result in "cardiac irregularities" sounded a lot better in discussions with other doctors and victims' families than saying "Prepulsid stops patient's hearts under some conditions and they die," which had been widely reported.

"We are asking doctors to conduct an ECG on the patient before giving it to patients. We sent out a letter on this topic to doctors in February."

I was devastated. Gloria was upstairs getting ready to join me at the funeral home. What about taking it off the market? I wondered. What about preparing full-page newspaper ads to warn patients? A definition of insanity is doing the same thing over and over and expecting different results.[2] What else could have happened except more deaths? Instead their response had been to fax out letters that apparently went unnoticed.

If eighty-one people had died in an air crash it would be on the front page of most major dailies in the free world and all over the TV news. There'd be a widely publicized investigation by an independent government agency—The National Transportation Safety Board. And there would be many follow-up stories. But for Johnson & Johnson and Health Canada, Prepulsid was just under discussion. There were no newspaper stories, no headlines, no photos at six. The victims probably died quietly in their homes or in a hospital bed. They might have been taking some other drug at the same time. Maybe they were quite sick. Were their deaths somehow insignificant, unimportant? Why were they not newsworthy? Had their deaths been in the media, maybe our doctors would have seen the story and warned us, or we might have read about them ourselves. Vanessa would be alive.

None of this made sense. A treatment that could be deadlier than what it treated. Numerous warnings that the doctors missed. And no one was surprised Vanessa died after reading the *CPS*. I don't know exactly when it dawned on me, but I feared this was business as usual. Vanessa was just the eighty-first victim—a statistic.

ECG (also EKG) stands for electrocardiogram—a test that measures important details of how your blood moves through your heart. The information from an ECG tells your doctor how your heart is working and that information can mean the difference between life and death. Telling doctors to order this test before prescribing Prepulsid would alert them that a stomach drug could adversely affect the heart. I wondered how many patients would take a drug for bloating that would require an ECG first. Some doctors would no doubt think back to Seldane, a drug for stuffy noses that could also kill patients. How could Johnson & Johnson actually think they could still ethically sell Prepulsid?

The more I learned, the more amazed I was that no risk had ever been mentioned to us—or to Vanessa. Either Gloria or

I attended all of her medical appointments with her. I was there when she was first prescribed Prepulsid over a year before. Her prescription had been renewed more than once, including the day she collapsed. No one ever mentioned an ECG. Gloria and I knew what ECG meant. I had that test years before as a precaution after suffering a migraine headache. Did Janssen-Ortho not have fax numbers for our doctors? Or did the doctors just not bother to read such warnings? And if they read them, what was the process in their office to contact all of their patients who were on that drug?

"We've had a concern," he said, "that some of the doctors apparently weren't reading the warnings."

If the family doctors weren't reading the warnings it obviously meant that Johnson & Johnson's customers were at risk. I assumed that any doctor who believed his patients are at risk must take action to correct the situation. All doctors are sworn to put patient welfare first, right? Their duty demands it. I had only been involved in prescription drug safety for fifteen minutes and it was pretty clear to me that the doctors weren't reading the safety warnings. It was inconceivable to me that none of the doctors had mentioned a word to a fifteen-year-old girl that has been taking the drug on and off for over a year. Surely *had they known* they would have said something. And here was a doctor who suspected some doctors were not reading the warnings. Yet instead of sympathizing with us, he was pointing the finger at his fellow doctors.

Dr. Barton explained how he thought Vanessa might have died. "QT prolongation is one aspect of cisapride (the generic name for Prepulsid). It shares a pathway with certain drugs, competing for the same process." I had no idea what he meant. I told him that Vanessa's problem was throwing up.

"Prepulsid is not efficacious and safe for bulimia. Bulimia is not a specific indication of the drug."

Although I didn't know what he meant at the time, "indi-cation" is a key medical-speak term. "Indication" means what the drug is supposed to do to your body and for which condition the regulators have approved it. Dr. Barton told me that Prepul-sid was "indicated" in the United States for nighttime dyspepsia. That means the U.S. Food and Drug Agency (FDA) had approved Prepulsid to be sold and prescribed in the U.S. for people who suffer heartburn at night. It was only legal for Johnson & Johnson to promote Prepulsid in the U.S. to people for that purpose.

In Canada, however, Prepulsid had been approved for three different conditions: gastroparesis, pseudo-obstruction and GERD. Gastroparesis—paralyzed stomach—normally occurs in patients with diabetes, kidney failure, or after surgery. Pseudo-obstruction occurs when food is not moving through one's digestive system. Either of these can cause bloating. GERD is gastroenterological reflux disease—what most people call heartburn.

Most important, Dr. Barton told me that in Canada and the U.S. Prepulsid was not approved for anyone who might be throwing up. He never mentioned fault. But he had given me two reasons which implied blame for Vanessa's death should be placed on her doctor. First, because he had diagnosed that she had a mild form of bulimia, Vanessa should not have been given Prepulsid at all. I could only assume the "Dear Doctor" letters explained that clearly. And second, he said Prepulsid shares a pathway and competes for the same process. I didn't learn fully what that meant for months. But I assumed he thought Vanessa had been taking another drug at the same time. Obviously this was very important, as the paramedics and doctors had all been asking about that after she collapsed. Other drugs in combination with Prepulsid could be danger-ous. I told him Vanessa had definitely not been taking any other drugs; that we didn't allow her to take anything more than Tylenol or ibuprofen.

"The prescribing information is pretty fierce for this drug," he said.

Fierce? I wondered, how? Four doctors seem to have missed that Prepulsid could be dangerous for patients that might be throwing up?

"There is no other drug to replace Prepulsid," he concluded. "Health Canada and the FDA see no reason to take it off the market."

This was all incredibly frustrating. I felt like shouting into the phone, "Instead of faxing out letters you idiots, why didn't you just pull the drug off the market? Why didn't you take out full-page ads in the newspapers or warn people? Why are you selling a drug that can kill patients to treat bloating and heartburn in the first place? No one ever died from heartburn or bloating. What in God's name is wrong with you people?"

I didn't shout at all. I simply ended the call. I suspected that everyone was going to be polite to the grieving father, and provide officially approved information. But no one was going to take responsibility for Vanessa's death.

I sat at my desk late that Monday morning gazing out at the school children coming home for lunch. Our appointment at the funeral home was in half an hour. I was numb inside. I've since read about the healing pattern of human grief. It comes in stages. Shock is first, with disbelief and numbness. I was still partially in that stage. And I still am. Part of me will be forever lost to numbness, as if I had lost a limb. Then follows denial: "I don't believe it. It can't really have happened." That took me weeks to get totally past. I don't remember when the harsh truth fully sunk in. Third is "bargaining"—when you make a deal with God—something like, "I'll be so good that maybe I'll wake up from this nightmare and find it's all a dream." This I experienced at the hospital the night Vanessa collapsed and night after night. But this was no bad dream. Guilt is supposed to be next and it sure was for me. I felt overwhelming guilt—a dark place where I spent hours and hours thinking "if only."

If only I had done some research on the Internet a month earlier.

If only we had chosen different doctors.

If only we had gone away for March break. It goes on and on. The next stage is supposed to be anger. And I thank God I had my wits about me. I realized I could simply not afford to get angry. Sure, friends and family would listen to me out of sympathy. But no one was going to believe an angry father. I had learned something that most people wouldn't want to believe, yet *must* believe to protect their own loved ones. Dangerous drugs were being given to our loved ones for non-life-threatening conditions. Many doctors don't know the dangers. Your families are not safe.

But if I was the angry father they'd never hear me. I'd be written off as too emotional, irrational; like the weeping parent on the TV news, quickly forgotten. On one side of this story would be the pathetic angry father, and on the other side the rational, self-controlled doctors or pharmacists who worked for Johnson & Johnson, and our own doctors—all in white lab coats with stethoscopes hanging around their necks, calmly rhyming off the medical-speak that sounds so indisputable. I knew if I became angry those responsible for Vanessa's death could get away with it. If I started shouting I might never find out how and why Vanessa had died. They'd win, and nothing would change. So I prayed for patience and resolve instead. I prayed to the same God that I felt had deserted me the night Vanessa had collapsed. I prayed for the strength to use the skills I had learned in business and politics to get to the bottom of Vanessa's death. Despite being consumed with a dreadful empty feeling, I had to remain in control. That morning sitting at my desk I quietly swore an oath to myself to find out what was responsible for her death, and expose the truth to help spare other families from going through what we were. I wasn't going to succumb to anger. But I was prepared to raise holy hell.

To provide some kind of justice for Vanessa, I knew I must keep my word.

Chapter 3

A Predictable Death

"Nearly all men die of their medicines, not of their diseases."
—J.B. Moliere, *Le Malade Imaginaire*

On September 13, 1999, John Calvert, aged forty-six, of Napa Valley, California, had suffered a heart attack. He'd been given some free samples of Prepulsid sixty-five days before by his doctor. The doctor was sued and settled with John's family for one hundred dollars. After a May 2003 trial that lasted eight weeks, the jury took three hours to decide that Prepulsid was not responsible for John's death. Janssen Pharmaceutical Inc., a division of Johnson & Johnson issued a press release saying it was "pleased" with the verdict.

**Monday, March 20, 2000
afternoon**

THAT WEEK IS PARTIALLY cloudy for me. Some things are crystal clear. Others are formless—as if they happened to someone else, not me. One thing I will never forget is that Vanessa's sister, Madeline, had decided on Monday morning that she would much rather be with her friends than at home sitting alone in the empty room she had shared with Vanessa, and courageously went to school. In class she logged on to the Internet and almost immediately found Janssen-Ortho's website and the "official prescribing information" for Prepulsid. In the small print was a sentence that said Prepulsid should not be given to patients who were throwing up. The combination could apparently cause a heart arrhythmia. Hearing this I was sickened. A seventeen-year-old student found in one minute what four experienced professionals apparently didn't bother to check over two years. One of them—our gastronenterologist—was an expert.

What Madeline had found on the web was the official drug label in the *CPS* that the doctors had read after she had collapsed. Every doctor has a copy in his or her office. And anyone could get onto the Internet and find it in a minute. This was the information that had eliminated the doctor's puzzlement—once they read it. It was logical to assume that had any of the doctors taken one minute to do the same thing as Madeline had in the previous weeks or months, her sister would be alive. They all knew that Vanessa had a problem with throwing up after meals. That was why she had gone to see them. This development broke open new wounds for us. The small print warning on the Prepulsid label meant Vanessa's death was not only preventable. It was predictable.

Tuesday, March 21, 2000
day two of our new life

The phone began to ring fairly steadily—neighbours and friends. Some called to find out if what they heard was really true. I told the story over and over. People brought prepared food and flowers. Their kindness was overwhelming. But no one could believe that a prescription drug had simply stopped the heart of the beautiful girl they had known at the Burl-Oak Canoe Club, or Oakville Trafalgar High School, or St. Jude's Church.

That morning I sat down in a daze to write Vanessa's obituary to be published in the *Globe and Mail*. I was trying in vain to sum up our child's life in three or four lines.[1] But before I did I made one more important call. I called the Government of Canada—Health Canada—to warn them about Prepulsid. I was connected with a doctor for the first of two conversations we had. By this time I was not surprised to hear that the people at Health Canada were aware of the risks related to Prepulsid as well.

"We are looking at it closely," he told me, "doing a very extensive review, and have been monitoring the situation in the U.S. as well."

"More discussion," I thought. He described the warning letters that had gone out to doctors as an interim step, to determine if the drug was safe or not. The last letter, dated February 25, 2000—directing doctors to do an ECG before prescribing Prepulsid—was not only faxed to ninety thousand doctors, but mailed to those who they could not confirm had received the fax. So Vanessa's doctors had probably all received the warning.

"I assure you," I told him patiently, "that Prepulsid is not safe. I'm in the process of planning my daughter's funeral. And she was taking no other drugs. Why don't you just order Prepulsid off the market?"

"We have no way to enforce a market withdrawal," he said. As a former MPP this shocked me. He was telling me the government of Canada had not given Health Canada the most important power it needed to protect its citizens from risky drugs.

I carefully controlled my voice, "What do you intend to do about it? There are thousands of people out there taking this stuff who don't know it could kill them. You should publish warnings in the newspapers. At least do a truly effective press release to warn people."

"That is not something Health Canada would do. That would be up to Johnson & Johnson. There is a concern that such warnings may frighten patients, and they'd stop taking their medication."

I didn't know whether to laugh or cry. If patients were frightened and stopped taking Prepulsid the worst outcome would be heartburn or bloating.

Incensed, I sat forward, and took a deep breath: "Has anyone ever died from *not* taking Prepulsid?"

"Not to my knowledge." he said without emotion. He promised to take my warning under advisement and continue their discussions. No such warnings ever came.

I've since found out our regulators almost always wait for the drug companies to issue safety warnings or remove their dangerous drugs off the market. Despite *forty-one* drugs being withdrawn from the Canadian market since the sixties, mostly for safety issues, there was no record that Health Canada had ordered any of them withdrawn. *Health Canada didn't even maintain a record of why the drugs had been withdrawn.*[2] Kind of like a police officer trying to persuade people to be good for decades, but making no arrests. And keeping no notes. The best example of why that is a dereliction of duty to the public is the worldwide withdrawal of Vioxx in November 2004. It wasn't the FDA or Health Canada that ordered this withdrawal. The FDA just held meeting after meeting until Merck finally decided to do it themselves. In the meantime between twenty-six to fifty-six thousand people on Vioxx had died from strokes and heart attacks.[3] This remains the greatest drug disaster in history—perhaps as many people dead as Americans died in the Vietnam War.

I wondered what would happen if the people who were responsible for checking jet aircraft tires or engines never ordered planes to be grounded because they weren't fit. Would the airlines negotiate with them instead? Would the airlines just send faxes to the pilots saying that they should be extra careful during takeoffs and landings? They should just test the engines and tires before each flight—like doing an ECG on patients.

When I was a member of Ontario's Provincial Parliament, a young man waiting at a bus stop in Oakville was hit by a spinning truck wheel that had fallen off a moving truck. He suffered terrible injuries. Others had died from flying truck wheels. Our government brought in strict new laws and heavy fines for having loose truck wheels and unsafe trucks on the road. We enforced the laws, placing roving inspection units on alternate routes that truckers took to avoid the regular inspection stations. And we actually put those trucks with loose wheels or poor brakes in truck "jail"—fenced-in areas where the trucks would be held until they were properly repaired. The Minister of Transportation, the late Al Palladini, ordered numerous press releases and posed for media photos to help warn truckers and alert the public. We didn't negotiate with truckers to keep unsafe trucks on the road. And the National Transportation Safety Board doesn't negotiate with airlines to keep unsafe aircraft in the air. What was wrong with the regulations at Health Canada? They were supposed to protect Vanessa.

Because of my oath I had to go public on what happened. Publicity was not going to be easy on any of us, but my goal was straightforward—to find the truth and warn others. Howard Mozel, a writer for one of our community papers, the *Oakville Beaver*, called and asked if he could interview me, as did Jim Polling from the *Hamilton Spectator*. I immediately agreed to both and invited them to our home. Other media outlets called. I talked to them all. It was surreal to be sitting in my own home giving interviews about how Vanessa died. It still felt like any moment she might walk into the room. "Hi, Dad. Mom and I are going to bake cookies. Want some?"

Sometimes I had unspoken conversations with Vanessa in my mind, and could hear her encouragement—telling me to warn others. I kept this to myself. People would think I'd lost it. Nevertheless the loss of privacy was hard on my family. In retrospect, the last thing they needed was to have journalists coming to the door. To this day I don't know if it was the right thing to do for them. It's what I had to do for Vanessa.

I began to get calls from neighbours. An infant three doors down had been on Prepulsid for spitting up. His father told me he'd checked the warning on the Internet and stopped giving him the drug. A mother from the Bronte area of Oakville called to say her teenage daughter had been taking Prepulsid while on a trip to Spain during school break, and was having frightening symptoms she described as "heart fluttering." She also stopped the drug as soon as they saw the *Oakville Beaver* article. "The story probably saved our daughter's life," she told me. One man told me his wife had suffered pains in her chest while taking Prepulsid and ended up in the hospital. She took the article from the *Oakville Beaver* to her doctor, who immediately took her off the drug and prescribed another drug to help her digest food.

This caught my attention because what I understood from Janssen-Ortho was that a key reason for keeping Prepulsid on the market was that there was no other drug to treat those patients. Apparently there was, at least in some cases.

But my local efforts seemed so hit and miss. I was wondering when officials at Johnson & Johnson and Health Canada were going to alert patients across Canada. Why was I, a grieving father, the only messenger about this risky drug?

Thursday, March 23, 2000
Vanessa's funeral

It was like acting in a play; making the funeral arrangements, greeting visitors, accepting flower deliveries, gifts of plants, and prepared food, and reading cards from well-wishers. Our friends and neighbours were very kind. Time seemed to stand still.

Several hundred well-wishers had visited the funeral home on Tuesday evening. Our respective family members stood beside us while Gloria and I greeted a long line of relatives, friends, and co-workers. When I think back to that evening it was like I had stepped outside myself and someone other than me was greeting the well-wishers—quite surreal. Strangely some people were so emotional that when they tried to console Gloria and me, we ended up consoling them. Two of my male friends— both fathers—attempted to greet me, but with tears forming in their eyes were totally unable to speak a word. Towards the end of the visitation I looked up to see my former boss, Premier Mike Harris, waiting in the line. It was kind of Mike to make time to drive out to Oakville to console us, but not a surprise. Mike is a dad too. I imagined all the fathers present—and mothers—were thinking the same thing. No matter how hard you try, sometimes you can't protect your children.

Over six hundred people came to Vanessa's funeral on Thursday morning. Archdeacon Alex Hewitt and the parishioners at St. Jude's were wonderful to us during this time. The choir members took time off work to provide beautiful choral music. Madeline and Hart were brave. Madeline chose the music for the service that Vanessa had loved to sing at choir school years before. I still can't listen to "I Vow to Thee My Country" which was sung to the tune of Holst's Jupiter, without a jolting and painful flashback to that day. It felt like we were in a heartbreaking movie. I kept thinking that such a wonderful service for

Vanessa, complete with a full church, should have been for her wedding day.

Vanessa was buried next to my father, Canon George Young of the Anglican Diocese of Toronto, at my mother's family burial place, the Massey Mausoleum at Mount Pleasant Cemetery, a beautiful arboretum in Toronto. When the graveside service was over two of Vanessa's best friends—Simone and Jen—travelled in a long limousine with us back to Oakville. We were all feeling quite numb having said goodbye to Vanessa, and yet remarkably full of her presence. She had loved to laugh with these girls, so when Simone suggested that it would be fun to take the limousine through the McDonald's drive-through window this ridiculous idea made perfect sense. Vanessa would have loved it. Ordering a Big Mac from the window of a funeral limousine. The limo was too long to get around the drive-through, so the girls just walked in to order, and laughed at the look on people's faces as we all got back in the limo. For a moment I could hear Vanessa's laughter as well. I remembered it later as if I was in slow motion: I turned my head, expecting to see her sitting there. I suppose I was going to tell her about this horrible long dream I'd had, now that she was back. I had other moments like that in the coming months.

The next day I got a call from my friend Lou Moska, another Oakville father.

"Terence, I just heard on the radio. Johnson & Johnson is pulling Prepulsid off the market in the U.S."

Johnson & Johnson was going to stop selling Prepulsid in the U.S. on July 14, 2000. I was relieved. Surely that would mean Johnson & Johnson would pull Prepulsid off the market in the 119 other countries it was sold, including Canada. Perhaps my phone calls had made a difference. I confess another reason I was relieved was that word spread quickly. The United States government had just validated the Young family's story.

After that we had no trouble convincing people of the risks. People knew now that what had happened in our family could happen in their family. They could take some action to protect themselves.

But I was to discover over the next few weeks that Johnson & Johnson weren't about to give up $90 million in Prepulsid sales in Canada that easily. Every day I waited to hear that Johnson & Johnson or Health Canada had finally pulled Prepulsid off the market in Canada. Apparently Johnson & Johnson had no intentions of taking Prepulsid off the market in Canada or apparently any country other than the United States. "There is no other drug to replace Prepulsid," is what Dr. Barton had said. And they had doctors convinced.

But there was another unspoken reason: I later read in a Johnson & Johnson annual report that despite the deaths, and despite taking Prepulsid off the open market in the U.S. Johnson & Johnson expected to still sell $250 million worth of Prepulsid worldwide that year. They would do this under a special access program they had negotiated in the U.S.: patients who felt the drug was helping them could apply through their doctor to obtain it. The millions of pills that were out there in their U.S. distribution chain could still bring in money. They would also do this by keeping Prepulsid on the market in Canada and as many as 117 other countries.

In April 2000 Prepulsid was still being prescribed and sold in Canada.

I watched every day for the public warnings in the newspapers. Nothing. By not backing down, Johnson & Johnson was stubbornly trying to keep up the facade in Canada that Prepulsid was safe enough. As if Canadians don't hear American news. I wondered if the people at Janssen Pharmaceutical, Johnson & Johnson's U.S. drug division, had even heard about Vanessa's death from their Canadian affiliate, Janssen-Ortho Canada. I assumed at first that the Johnson & Johnson March 23 announcement to withdraw Prepulsid was to save patient lives.

Sadly, this was naive.

I discovered that Vanessa's death had nothing to do with it. Three months before, a nine-month-old infant, Gage Stevens, had died in his sleep after being given Prepulsid with Tagamet (which reduces stomach acid) for spitting up, as part of a clinical trial out of Pittsburgh Children's Hospital. The Pittsburgh Coroner had blamed his death on SIDS (sudden infant death syndrome).[4] But Gage's mother, an operating room nurse, had heard rumours about Prepulsid and didn't accept that conclusion. The form she had signed to enrol Gage in the drug trial had stated that Prepulsid was FDA-approved for children. In fact it was not.

By the time Gage had started on Prepulsid, eighteen children under nineteen years old taking Prepulsid had died. Two months after Gage's death the coroner changed Gage's death certificate to say he died of heart arrhythmia—a known side-effect of Prepulsid with Tagamet.

Johnson & Johnson was facing an FDA meeting in Washington on April 12, 2000, where experts would discuss what to do about Prepulsid. A clear possibility was an FDA order to pull Prepulsid off the market. But the stakes were far bigger than U.S. sales. Prepulsid was a "blockbuster" drug—selling over $1 billion a year in 119 countries. Many of these countries relied on underfunded and understaffed regulatory bodies that simply copied FDA orders. If Johnson & Johnson waited for an FDA order to stop selling Prepulsid in the U.S., it might start a chain reaction of regulatory orders worldwide to stop selling Prepulsid. On the other hand, by announcing they were withdrawing Prepulsid "voluntarily" in the U.S. they would avoid a direct FDA order to withdraw Prepulsid, and help the company to keep it on the market elsewhere. Johnson & Johnson is still selling Prepulsid in many countries today through its many subsidiaries.

I learned there were over 2,600 SIDS deaths in North America in 2000, each one a mystery. Prepulsid was being prescribed to thousands of infants for spitting up. Drug-induced long QT can stop an infant's heart and be mistakenly categorized as a SIDS death. Naturally I wondered how many other SIDS deaths might have been due to long QT caused by Prepulsid.

Not withdrawing Prepulsid in Canada was just morally wrong to me. Canadians deserve the same protection as Americans. If Prepulsid was not safe enough for Americans, what about other unsuspecting patients across the world?

In the weeks following Vanessa's death I watched Gloria, Madeline, and Hart attempt to get back to some form of new normal. Gloria went back to work fundraising at St. Peter's Hospital Foundation in Hamilton. Madeline and Hart went back to school—all trying to adjust to the fact that life can be incredibly unjust. Meanwhile they watched me struggling for some kind of justice—by determining who was responsible for our loss. It must have been hard on them. I suppose it wasn't the sanest way to spend my time. I'm no Ralph Nader. But I had to keep my word.

In April, I resumed development of my government relations business. I had a small office in a lawyer's building in downtown Oakville. A few months before, a lawyer I knew—Jeremy Taylor[5]—had kindly offered me some vacant space free for a few months to establish my business, after which I began paying rent. I planned to spend two hours every day on my research on Prepulsid, and the rest on business. But the information I found became overwhelming and by mid-April I was spending half my time on research. During the day I prospected for new clients, attending as many events as I could, handing out business cards. I landed a few. I helped a high-tech printing company find new business and was asked to assist St. Peter's

Hospital in Hamilton—where Gloria worked—at Queen's Park. Between daytime business duties, and in the evenings, I continued my research. There was still no official warning in Canada about Prepulsid, and I felt as if I was the only one that was going to pursue this issue to its conclusion—whatever that would be.

One day in early April a friend from the insurance industry invited me to lunch. The conversation quickly came around to how my family and I were doing. I told him we were all still feeling shell-shocked.

"You have to sue," he told me bluntly. "It's a no-brainer. The impact of the trauma you and your family suffered will stay with you. This is not the same as an accidental death, especially with you all there. It's the only way to even get the attention of those responsible." He gave me the name and number of a top litigation lawyer. "You've got a strong case."

We talked about it some more and I thanked him.

But I really didn't know if I had a legal case at all. I had to find out exactly what the warnings said. I began to call doctors and others I had met in the drug industry when I had been an MPP.

In April I spoke with almost twenty family physicians, some of whom I'd known for decades. A few said they just didn't use Prepulsid in their practice. Some of them commented vaguely that they had "seen something in the past" but that was it. They couldn't remember if it was a faxed letter or article in a medical journal. What shocked me was they couldn't remember what the warnings said. Only one of them knew the true risks of Prepulsid before Johnson & Johnson's last warning letter in February. That was my cousin Dr. David Knox, a family physician in Orangeville, Ontario.

David told me Prepulsid was first introduced as a replacement for Maxeran but with no "oculogyric crisis." I noticed that even the most caring doctors sometimes use medical-speak, forgetting that most people simply don't know what their words mean. I looked up "oculogyric crisis" after the call. Sure enough, Maxeran (metoclopramide), also known as Reglan, had been sold for bloating. It had some rare but disgusting side effects: an oculogyric crisis is an uncontrollable muscle spasm of the eye, mouth or tongue. One elderly woman had apparently suffered a reaction to Maxeran that made her tongue stick out—permanently. Sometimes patients' eyes get stuck in one position, like straight up, and they can't move them until the drug wears off. Or their mouth stays wide open. Maxeran could also rarely cause life-threatening reactions: anxiety, violence or "depersonalization." The list of Maxeran side effects made me feel a little sick.

David was straightforward. "I don't trust new drugs and don't prescribe them for patients until they've been on the market for ten to fifteen years. Then I look at their track record." Why was this the first time I'd ever heard this approach?

"How can you remember what's safe and what isn't?" I asked.

"There is no way you can keep up with them all. The proliferation of new drugs is massive. I use a small number of drugs that I know well. Anything else I would use only after reading up on it carefully. When there is a warning, I just stop prescribing the drug. My own understanding is that Prepulsid was contraindicated for bulimia."

I told David I wasn't sure Vanessa had bulimia, but she had the most prominent symptom—throwing up. I know her doctors thought so. But I had learned that bulimia has four components: binge eating; the use of laxatives or diuretics; throwing up; and "no other eating disorder." We never had laxatives or diuretics in the house, and Vanessa was not a binge eater. She had no other eating disorder. Nevertheless, I told him that throwing up had bothered her on and off for over a year. That was why she had seen the doctors.

I'd heard the word "contraindicated" before and looked it up after the call. Contraindication comes from two words put together—contra and indicated. It means against the approved use. It's a huge red flag. Contraindication refers to two (or more) things mixed together in your system that can be truly dangerous: another drug, or a condition—like throwing up, or even a food. I had never heard that a food eaten with a drug might be dangerous. The most common one is ordinary grapefruit juice. Ordinary grapefruit juice consumed with any one of a long list of drugs could possibly stop your heart. There are at least two reported deaths of men in the U.S. related to this—one with Seldane, now off the market, and one with the world's best-selling drug—Lipitor.[6]

David told me he did not prescribe Prepulsid, referring to a letter about it in the *New England Journal of Medicine* in 1996. I was impressed. Here was a family doctor that read medical journals, and remembered an article from four years before. Then he asked me if Dr. Kayner had told our doctor that Vanessa's problem was throwing up. "Of course," I said "That was the only reason she went to see her."

He was silent for a moment, then said: "There's a huge difference between contraindication and 'outside the indications' or off-label use. It's very dangerous to prescribe anything 'contra' the indications. It's the doctor's responsibility to know the dangers."

But our doctor was a specialist. Did she have better information than the other doctors I wondered? And what did it matter, considering the result? I was incensed. "I don't want to destroy anyone's career, but things have to change. I've been advised to file a lawsuit."

"Any doctor can make a mistake. But a lawsuit could provide some benefit to the system. It could save someone's life."

God, I felt guilty. If David had been our family doctor, Vanessa would be alive. But Orangeville was an hour and a half away. Orangeville, Ontario, a farming community of thirty thousand, had this knowledgeable doctor who carefully protected his patients against adverse drug reactions; and Oakville, with one of the highest average incomes in Canada, had at least four doctors who'd never put it together. I thanked David for his time.

Dr. Garnet Maley was in nearby Milton. I'd met him at one or two political functions when I was an MPP, a nice man. He told me Johnson & Johnson had marketed Prepulsid aggressively in the nineties. Only in the last month or two had he heard about the warnings. There was an alternative drug for patients with bloating that had an established safety record—Motilium. Another alternative to Prepulsid! Even if Maxeran (metoclopramide) had some ugly side effects, maybe Motilium was safer.[7]

Dr. Albert Schumacher, then president of the Ontario Medical Association, shed some light on this. "I used Prepulsid in my practice," he said, "and Motilium before that, another Johnson & Johnson drug. I remember when Prepulsid was being marketed because I connect it to the same time Baghdad was being bombed" (the first Gulf War in January 1991).

That really puzzled me. "Why would Johnson & Johnson introduce a new drug which would compete with an effective one they were already selling?" I asked him.

"They marketed it as being more efficacious at the time. But they also had new patent life for Prepulsid. Motilium was coming off patent." This was my first lesson in drug marketing. He was referring to Johnson & Johnson's business plan to introduce Prepulsid to retain their customers that used Motilium. I've researched this practice at length. Exclusive patent rights are granted to new molecules (drugs) in Canada for twenty years. But by the time a patented drug goes through testing and approvals, and gets on the market, there might only be twelve years left of exclusive rights to make and sell it. In the late eighties, Johnson & Johnson's Motilium was running out of exclusive selling time. By introducing a new patented drug for the same symptoms—Prepulsid for bloating—Johnson & Johnson could prevent some loss of customers to generic copies. As I would soon discover, this is quite common in the drug industry. The problem is that the second drug is not necessarily better than the first, nor as safe. It is however, more profitable. I asked Dr. Schumacher if he'd heard of a drug data company I'd been told about called IMS.[8]

"Yes. Half or more of the big pharma companies use IMS. They track prescription use by doctor, and target what they call 'high-scrip' doctors. But in British Columbia they passed a law against it."[9] I was pleased to hear that. I still didn't know why Dr. Kayner thought Prepulsid would be safe for Vanessa. The idea that a drug sales rep (detail rep) can track what prescriptions doctors wrote was unsettling. I was to learn over time that doctors don't even track the prescriptions they write.[10] And prescribing information is private professional information. Knowing what doctors prescribe would give the drug sales reps an upper hand in persuading the doctor to prescribe their drugs.

"When did you first hear of any risks from Prepulsid?" I asked Dr. Schumacher.

"I stopped prescribing it when it was pulled off the U.S. market in March. I was shocked at this withdrawal. We were using this stuff like candy." I assume he was speaking for his peer group—family physicians.

Immediately I thought of what Dr. Eggar had said the night Vanessa had collapsed. "They dish it out like water." That night is still clear in my mind. I called his office and left a message.

Dr. Eggar is a pediatric cardiologist. He specializes in treating children's hearts. Although he did not conduct the autopsy, if anyone would know what really happened to Vanessa, I suspected it would be he. He was kind enough to return my call the same day, and verified what Dr. Schumacher had said. "We were dispensing it like water. G.I. people use it a lot [referring to Gastro-Intestinal specialists—stomach doctors]. I've had no trouble with it because I use it according to the manufacturer's instructions—with the indications. If there was any potential electrolyte problem I would stay away."

Then Dr. Eggar reflected on how he thought Vanessa died. "With Vanessa we have a theory, but we may not be able to prove it.[11] We assume it had to do with electrolyte abnormalities. Low potassium is high-risk for cardiac rhythms. Isuprel and magnesium had started her heart in the hospital. Torsade waves showed on her strip. Cisapride [Prepulsid] is one of the few things that cause torsades."

Over the next few days I read everything I could about the human heart. The heart emits electrical signals to cause contractions. These signals can be recorded on an ECG test in a "waveform" on a strip of paper. That was the "strip" Dr. Eggar referred to. It's a common test and was the one he used in the hospital when he was trying to revive Vanessa. Different parts of this waveform are assigned letters in order: P, Q, R, S, and T. The QT interval is the time it takes for activation and inactivation of the heart's lower chambers—the ventricles. This interval is measured in thousandths of a second, and if it takes longer than normal it's called a prolonged QT interval. Or long QT. When that happens a rapid heartbeat can occur called torsades de pointes. That means the heart can't contract effectively, and the normal amount of blood is reduced to the body and brain. If the heart can't recover its normal rhythm it may spasm and go into ventricular fibrillation, like an engine misfiring. Without immediate medical intervention— emergency action to get the person's heart started—death can follow within minutes. All this happens more often when the patient's electrolytes are low because the electrical signals can't be conducted without potassium and magnesium. Electrolytes can be depleted when a person throws up repeatedly or has diarrhea.

Dr. Eggar continued: "Low potassium also makes prolonged QT worse. This is high risk for cardiac arrhythmias."

So Prepulsid probably caused long QT in Vanessa's heart, and low electrolytes might have made her QT phase longer—causing a deadly heart arrhythmia. *That's why Prepulsid was contraindicated for throwing up.* And that's why it was critical for doctors to get a truly effective warning.

Does she [Vanessa] have long QT? That was the question I'd been asked that in the emergency room that night. Well, some people have long QT as a condition—congenital long QT. It can he inherited from your parents. It can show up as fainting spells during periods of high emotion—fright, anger or pain—or during exercise. Usually, a child with long QT will have fainting spells before age ten. Some of the sudden deaths that you hear about amongst young people while playing sports are caused by congenital long QT. They might have had no idea they had it, having missed any warning signals. I felt sure Vanessa did not. We have no family history of long QT, and the only time Vanessa ever felt faint in her life was about a year before at a sleepover while she had been taking Prepulsid. Because we had no Prepulsid warning, we thought at the time her fainting was caused by low blood sugar when she stood up quickly. Yet another thing I felt guilty about: a missed warning sign for Prepulsid.

I asked Dr. Eggar about Motilium.

"Motilium works."

I told him the Prepulsid label said not to give Prepulsid to patients who were throwing up. "Why didn't the doctors see that caution?"

"It was not a clear warning. Only in the last few months did I get clear warnings. But I work in a branch of medicine where we are very aware of long QT. The average family physician or GI doctor [stomach specialist] does not pay very close attention to the stuff. The Prepulsid label was vague."

I thanked Dr. Eggar for his help.

But was Vanessa given Prepulsid inappropriately because the warnings and label were vague, or because the doctors didn't read them? I knew I had to study the warnings and labels carefully, and talk to industry insiders. But I had a more urgent task: to make sure this death wasn't swept under the rug. I was on the right track in learning how Vanessa died. It was going to be a lot tougher discovering who was responsible.

Chapter 4

A Conspiracy of Silence

"'But I don't want to go among mad people,' Alice remarked.
'Oh. You can't help that' said the Cat: 'we're all mad here.'"
—Alice's Adventures in Wonderland

April 2000

HALTON REGIONAL POLICE had launched a routine investigation into Vanessa's death, and the results would go to the
regional coroner. A young police investigator carefully interviewed me and other witnesses. But I didn't think one investigator would have the time to unravel the complex issues I'd
uncovered. I knew to prevent similar deaths we needed a coroner's inquest—an open process on the public record. We also
needed a jury to hear the expert evidence that I'd heard. In May
I called the office of the Chief Coroner for Ontario James Young
(no relation to me) to brief him. The next day Deputy Chief
Coroner Jim Cairns called me back.

"Inquests are not automatic." he explained. "If it appears

that an inquest might be necessary to save other lives the odds are better of getting one."

I did my utmost to persuade him. "Based on what I've learned about the safety warnings I believe an inquest would save lives, by showing who was to blame."

"Inquests do not assign blame," he cautioned me. "The jury at an inquest does not determine guilt. They determine a cause of death, and make recommendations to change the system to prevent similar deaths."

Fine, I thought. We'll start with the cause. That will no doubt shine a light on who was to blame. Jim also told me there had been another death of a teenage girl related to Prepulsid in the Toronto area, but it was not clear-cut like Vanessa's case.

"Vanessa's was a 'clean' death. Since it appears that no other drugs were involved and she had no other health issues, it will help us isolate the cause of death."

The coroners were pleased: They had a clean death. I had never thought of death as clean before. Jim chaired the coroners' Pediatric Review Committee that met monthly to discuss trends and other cases. He told me they had been concerned about Prepulsid's adverse reactions. "All the experts on the committee agree that it should not be handed around like Smarties."

Because Vanessa died in Hamilton, Dr. David Eden, the regional coroner for Niagara and Hamilton, would decide if we'd get an inquest. The publicity might just get the attention of officials at Health Canada and the Johnson & Johnson executives in New Jersey. But could we get one? On May 27, 2000, I wrote to Dr. Eden to make a formal request.

I felt like I had fallen down the rabbit hole. It seemed that everyone in authority had known Prepulsid was a risky drug, but never told the people taking it—or the doctors giving it to them. And I was worried that time might run out for other girls or infants still on Prepulsid whose parents didn't read the papers.

So I called Dr. Eden in Hamilton to plead with him to order Health Canada to issue a public warning.

"I have notified Health Canada," he told me. "They don't have a causal link and can't issue a warning yet. There are grounds for concern."

Whoa. That's not what I had heard. *My* understanding was that Prepulsid was pulled off the U.S. market by Johnson & Johnson because the body count was too high. Besides, what possible harm could come from issuing a warning to patients? God, it was frustrating. What ever happened to "better safe than sorry?" I thought. Dr. Eden tried to placate me. "Generally, U.S. removal is followed by Canadian removal."

Good, I thought, when?

He referred me to Dr. Ken Ockenden in his office, who was in charge of Vanessa's case. His mandate was to find the facts and make recommendations to prevent further deaths now, even before an inquest. We connected by phone.

"The autopsy and preliminary report are complete," Ken told me. "No other drugs were found in Vanessa's blood other than what was given to her in the hospital after she collapsed. And there was no anatomic cause of death."

That meant Vanessa had a healthy body; no surprise to me, but nevertheless a huge relief. Honestly, I had lost my faith in doctors, and I was fearful someone might make another mistake. And there were no other drugs in her blood before she collapsed. But there was still a potential escape hatch for Prepulsid. I was fearful about what Dr. Eggar had said about congenital long QT. All the coroner had to say was that Vanessa showed some sign of congenital long QT and it would be all over. Her death would be meaningless. I asked Dr. Ockenden about it.

"Vanessa had no heart abnormalities," he said. "The next step is to send blood samples to the Centre for Forensic Sciences in Toronto to get a toxicology report." Toxic means poison.

Toxicology is detecting poisons. The lab would do a microscopic examination to verify if Prepulsid poisoned Vanessa.

I was pleased then immediately consumed with guilt. I had no business feeling pleased about a "clean" death. Yet this was a crucial step. With no family history or evidence of congenital long QT, the escape hatch for those responsible could be closed. But the more I'd learned, the more I felt sure that issuing a warning about Prepulsid was not enough.

"Would the toxicology report be enough to establish this causal link that Health Canada wants before they order Prepulsid off the market?" I asked.

"With a normal heart and no other drugs in her blood, the presence of cisapride [Prepulsid] would be cause and effect."

Good. That was the first time I'd heard the term "cause and effect." I resolved to learn exactly what it meant. But there was a problem: The toxicology report could take two to four months. So I made a call to John Guthrie, chief of staff to Solicitor General David Tsubouchi, who had authority over inquests and explained the urgency of the lab report. He promised to get back to me.

One of the people I met with had contacted me shortly after the funeral to express his sympathies—Alex Demerse.[1] Alex had worked inside the international drug industry for years, for more than one major pharmaceutical company.

I had always liked Alex. I found him to be forthright, frank, and knowledgeable. He was also a father, and other parents had been particularly helpful to me during this time. I suspect they were thinking, "What if this was me?" I hoped Alex would give me the insider perspective.

It was a sunny weekday afternoon in mid-April when I pulled up in front of Alex's beautiful home and rang the bell. We had the house to ourselves as we sat down in his living room. We talked a little about our families briefly, and then I jumped right

in: "Alex, we had absolutely no warning of any risks of Prepulsid. She was taking no other drug. How could this happen?"

Alex had been following Vanessa's case in the media. I will
never forget what he told me next. It was like taking a cold
shower. He sat forward on the edge of his chair, energized as he
launched into his detailed answer:

"They knew. It became a dollar sign for them. They were
selling a billion dollars' a year of Prepulsid. These big drug
companies weigh deaths against billions of dollars. Janssen-
Ortho marketed this drug to become the drug of choice. The
whole industry is about marketing blockbusters—drugs that sell
over a billion dollars a year. For example, ten deaths versus two
billion in sales is no contest. From the industry view it's better
to keep selling it if the lawsuits are minimal—especially in
Canada. If they lose any lawsuits they appeal the decision or
settle with the families. It's just a cost of doing business."

Clearly Alex wasn't holding back. I sat quietly taking notes,
briefly interjecting questions.

"Why especially in Canada?"

"Because in Canada there are very few drug liability lawsuits
compared to the United States. And even if they are sued and lose,
the maximum damages a drug company would have to pay in
Canadian courts for a death of a child are small, maybe fifty to a
hundred thousand dollars. That's nothing to them. They'd spend
multiples of that on a free trip for their top sales reps. And it's
very hard to beat them I court. Proving adverse drug reactions is
based on probabilities, and they always have studies geared to
push some information aside. The system is flawed."

In fairness, Alex wasn't picking on Johnson & Johnson or
their drug division, Janssen-Ortho. He was talking about the
international drug companies as a group—the world's biggest.
He was talking about them as all being the same—the same
methods, the same ethics. I was being briefed not just on one

company, but an international industry. And I've seen since that the major international pharmaceutical companies—referred to as Big Pharma—do share most of their business practices. Since the nineties, the industry has become notorious for takeovers, collaborations, and buyouts, so names and players change, but so far key business practices have not.

"Why haven't I heard these things before?" I asked Alex. I was no recluse. I had been in public life, and currently worked in government relations. I read media clippings from forty newspapers daily and many periodicals. I made my living on information. He was shaking his head in agreement.

"When the pharmaceutical companies settle out of court, they make the families sign secret agreements that they will never talk publicly about the drug or the death again. Otherwise, no deal. If the families talk about it, they'll be sued to get the money back. The victims' families are basically sworn to secrecy."

"But what about legal fees? And their public image? Don't the companies care about that?"

He shook his head. "Ironically, the cost of legal fees *helps* them, because they have such deep pockets. It's David versus Goliath. Most victims settle out of court because they can't face the huge risk of losing, or being ordered to pay a half-million dollars for the drug company's legal costs. Who can risk half a million dollars to win $100,000? And lawyers in Canada won't take on a case like that without money upfront. Most people can't afford it. Besides, grieving families are emotionally devastated and want closure. If not, the drug company lawyers just keep fighting them until they wear them down. It can take years. The families give up. So the cases rarely get to court."

"Still," I said. "The companies could lose a lot of money in some of the American class actions."

"They can *afford* to lose. They make billions. It's a cost of doing business. They put it right in their business plans. Anyway, they *buy insurance* against huge settlements. If a drug starts killing patients and they lose in court, the insurance will cover most of the costs."

I was disgusted, yet fascinated at the same time. If the drug companies could buy insurance against harming or killing patients, that would explain their lack of caution. But where was accountability? I was thinking that I could never be part of a cover-up like that. An inquest would hopefully expose how Vanessa died—but to keep my word I would have to expose who was responsible. A courtroom trial seemed the only way.

"Are you saying I shouldn't sue them?" I asked.

He raised his arms excitedly, palms open. "No. Your case is different. You have grounds for a major lawsuit. First, there are already eighty known deaths. And in Vanessa's case they can't do what drug companies usually do—blame it on another drug. Because there wasn't one. Nor was there an overdose or serious illness. Their usual defenses are gone. What they will try to do is to blame it on the doctors. You should sue them as well."

It was hard to imagine companies being so wealthy.

"The markup on drugs must be high."

"They are huge. The big international drug companies are the most profitable companies in the world. They might spend maybe three hundred million to develop each new patented drug, but when sales exceed three hundred million those costs are covered. That can happen in a few years. They have years after that to make profits. Once they have recovered the initial R&D [research and development] costs, their only costs are the cost of making powder, packaging the pills, and marketing them. The markups on prescription drugs are in the hundreds of per cent. Sometimes in the thousands. It's like a licence to print money. And they avoid taxes like crazy. They own subsidiaries in tax havens like Ireland or Puerto Rico that make the powders by the ton—literally. You can make three million pills from a ton of powder. They buy the powder from companies *they own* at a huge markup, so they can show their drug costs are high when our governments are paying for them. It's called transfer pricing. They transfer the transaction—and the profits—to jurisdictions with no taxes, or low taxes. And the market price of a drug has nothing to do with what it costs to develop or produce the drug. They charge what the market will bear. If patients or the government will pay a hundred dollars a month for a drug, that's what they'll charge. If they'll pay thirty thousand dollars a year, that's what they'll charge."

I told him about the four warning letters sent out to doctors. He was shaking his head side to side as I spoke.

"But the companies *know* they don't read them. Doctors are very busy people. After seeing forty or fifty patients doctors don't sit down at the end of the day and read a big pile of faxes. The drug companies issue warnings instead of pulling the drug off the market. They keep sales climbing, while protecting themselves against lawsuits. That's how you create a blockbuster."

This was so hard to believe. "How do they know the doctors don't read them?"

He shrugged his shoulders and turned his palms up. "Some do. But most don't. The companies know that because after issuing warning letters the sales keep going up! A few years back, Prepulsid was not a huge seller. Janssen then started heavily marketing it, making it the drug of choice. Now it's a blockbuster. But people had already died after taking it."

I told him how easily Madeline had found the warning regarding throwing up. "What about the drug label?" I asked. "Four doctors didn't notice that Prepulsid was not supposed to be given to anyone who was throwing up."

Alex leaned forward to make sure I didn't miss a word. "Labels aren't written for doctors. They are written for lawyers, *by* lawyers, to protect the drug companies against lawsuits. In some cases the drug sales reps even tell doctors: 'Don't worry about the label. That's just lawyers being extra careful. This drug is safe.' The warnings are in small print so the doctors and patients won't read them and stop using the drug. Labels are also pages long, sometimes forty pages or more, making the safety information too time-consuming to find. Even doctors don't understand the risks. But if the companies get sued, they can point to the small print and blame the doctors."

I remembered Madeline saying she had to zip through a few Internet pages to find the warning. But she was looking for a warning. If you weren't, I imagined it could have been easy to miss. I had to conclude doctors don't look for warnings.

"The labels are different in the U.S. and Canada," I said. "How can a drug become a blockbuster when it's approved for different conditions in different countries?"

"Easy. A lot of the sales are off-label."

I'd heard this term before. It means the drug is prescribed to treat symptoms for which it has never been officially proven safe. Doctors prescribe off-label all the time. For example, Prepulsid was never approved as safe and effective for children. And Dr. Barton had mentioned that throwing up was not a specific "indication" of Prepulsid. Yet doctors had commonly experimented with it off-label in treating bulimic teens! So, beyond the obvious issue that Prepulsid sometimes stopped hearts, Vanessa's condition and age were two more reasons Vanessa should have not been given Prepulsid. I was counting.

"If it's only legal to promote a drug for its approved use," I asked, "How does it get up to blockbuster status?"

"That's easy. The gatekeepers. Our doctors. Doctors are allowed to prescribe drugs for whatever they want. They are like gods. The detail reps (sales reps) are supposed to provide doctors with the details about new drugs. What they do is push their latest drug, giving the doctors all the information that makes their drug look good, while knocking their competitor's drugs. This is all verbal of course. There's nothing in writing. And they might mention that so-and-so, a leading expert, uses their drug off-label on patients with another condition. And it helps the patients."

"Isn't that illegal promotion?"

"Absolutely, but try and catch them. Remember, nothing goes in writing."

"What if the doctor calls that expert and he denies what the detail rep claimed?"

"That's unlikely. The expert is probably on the drug company payroll in one way or another. He may have made speeches or conducted a clinical study for the drug company. The companies pay between five and twenty thousand dollars per patient enrolled in a study. There are lots of different ways they get money into doctor's pockets. The specialist named by the drug rep is going to say good things about the drug."

I quickly did the math. A study with one hundred patients could potentially pay a specialist two million dollars. I wondered if any of Vanessa's doctors ever received money for research from Johnson & Johnson.

"Do the patients know if their doctor is receiving drug company money on the side?"

"Usually not. There is no statute that requires doctors to tell the patients their doctor has a potential conflict of interest. Sometimes the doctors set up their own foundations for the cheques to be made out to. Then they draw a salary."

This stunned me. Doctors could earn as much as two million dollars on the side by testing a drug on their patients, and aren't required to tell them they are getting thousands of dollars to do it? I imagined a doctor with a trusting elderly lady sitting before him with high blood pressure. He could prescribe an older drug approved by our regulators with a proven safety profile. Or he could prescribe the drug that is not proven safe and effective to treat high blood pressure—but that he is being paid twenty thousand dollars per patient to study. All he'd have to do is tell the patient that he's prescribing a new use of a known drug for her as part of a trial and that he thinks will work better: "Is that OK?" Which drug will he choose? And what if his study was almost complete, and if some patients on the experimental drug told him they want to stop because it makes them feel strange? That might set his study—and payday—back six months. What would he do? Would he persuade a patient that was telling him he'd had an adverse reaction to keep taking the drug . . . for the greater good of mankind?

When I was first elected as MPP I had to complete and sign a disclosure statement for the Integrity Commissioner of Ontario declaring everything I owned of value—all property, investments and directorships. That became public information. And no MPP is allowed to accept gifts of any kind associated with their position, other than things like ceremonial presentations. That's how strict the conflict of interest rules are for politicians in Ontario. Yet somehow doctors—who have power over life and death—are allowed to secretly accept hundreds of thousands of dollars on the side, while putting their patients at risk.

"What if the doctors don't buy the sales pitches?" I asked.

"The companies don't waste time on doctors who don't pay attention or write a lot of prescriptions. They focus on high prescribers—the ones who write fifty to a hundred prescriptions a day. They're called high-scrip docs and the industry loves them. The drug companies buy the doctors' prescribing information from data companies like IMS, who collect it from the pharmacies. Then the reps target these high-scrip docs—visit them regularly, provide lots of free samples, take them out to dinner, whatever it takes to build a relationship. They track how their pitches have done the next month."

This reminded me how Las Vegas casinos treat their "high rollers," the "fish" so big they call them "whales." Lots of free hospitality—as long as they keep playing.

"So they would have a good idea when their sales pitch for off-label use is working by the sales figures?"

"Yes, but not just that. They go back and *ask* the doctor. Did you try this drug for the other use? Did it help your patients? Will you prescribe it more often?"

"Why do the doctors put up with these intrusions? Don't they realize how biased the detail reps are?"

"A lot of reasons. There are too many drugs to track— over twenty thousand including over-the-counter (OTC) drugs. No doctor could keep track of them all, and new ones are approved every week. In most medical schools doctors don't get any formal courses on pharmacology—how drugs work in the body—so they are not well equipped to argue with the detail reps who come in armed with slick pamphlets full of colour graphs and endorsements from leading specialists, as well as gifts and free samples. The doctors are also busy. If they can grab lunch or use an evening out at a fine restaurant to learn about new drugs, why not? Especially since the detail reps pay the shot."

I couldn't help wondering if any of Vanessa's doctors had spent time with the Janssen-Ortho detail reps and I imagined how the conversation might have gone: "Oh, by the way it's effective for teens that throw up."

"Why doesn't the government act to change the system?" I asked Alex.

He raised his arms up excitedly. "These companies have more money than many countries, and unlimited money for lawyers. They'll take on governments and win. Even the U.S. government, the FDA. They usually fight first, and then settle quietly later. Besides, they have very influential lobbyists, and huge budgets for political donations. They usually get what they want in Washington, and Ottawa."

I immediately felt guilty. When I was an MPP I had been part of this system. Lobbyists from Big Pharma invited me to golf tournaments, or black-tie dinners. And they bought tickets to my fundraisers. We got along very well. I listened to their pitches out of courtesy and they were quite convincing. One of them later brought his PowerPoint slide show to my office to explain how their bone-loss drug reduced hip fractures in older women and saved the government money in reduced hospital stays. Of course the figures were all rosy guesstimates and he never mentioned the cost of treating the women who suffered adverse reactions.

I changed the subject. "How could so many adverse reactions be ignored? Health Canada still hasn't taken Prepulsid off the market. How can they just do nothing?"

"It's worse than you think. Only a small percentage of adverse reactions are reported. It's a huge problem, because adverse reaction reporting by doctors is voluntary. There are probably hundreds more adverse reactions to Prepulsid than the official figures indicate, maybe thousands. Doctors report maybe one per cent of adverse reactions."

This was incredible to me. I spent weeks trying to verify this from the most reliable sources. Every study I could find backed Alex up.[2] For example, in 1993 former FDA Commissioner David Kessler, later associate director of safety, estimated in the *Journal of the American Medical Association* that fewer than one per cent of all doctors report injuries and deaths following the administration of prescription drugs.

My mind was racing. This could mean that many more people had died from Prepulsid. "Why don't they report them?"

"They're afraid of being sued! What doctor wants to sit down at the end of a long day and fill out a form for the government that says he almost killed a patient? And sometimes they just can't tell if it was an adverse reaction or not. Time is also a problem. Most doctors have patients waiting at any given time all day."

Now I was on the edge of my chair. "The doctors don't report the adverse reactions to the regulators or drug companies. So the drug labels only show about one per cent of the reactions that actually happen. Then other doctors read the label and think the drug is quite safe."

"Right. It's great for sales. But it's bad for patients. The doctors who do look at the drug labels might notice that a drug had been given to a million patients and been related to six deaths. That could be six very sick people, or six older people taking ten drugs at a time. Or patients with other conditions. Most doctors would not be alarmed at this figure. But if it read ten times that, sixty deaths, or one hundred times that, six hundred, that would be a huge red flag for doctors."

"Has Health Canada has ever ordered the drug companies to publish more accurate estimated numbers of adverse reactions on their labels?"

He laughed. "No. The whole system is based on figures they all know are way too low." I sat back exhausted. I was literally seeing the world in a different way.

"So who in the system is acting totally to protect patients?"

Alex paused. Briefly his eyes seemed to be searching the far corners of the room. I could tell he was scanning his own memory. "No one," he replied in resignation. "It's all about money."

I drove home feeling overwhelmed. This thing was like peeling an onion. First it was doctors not reading the warnings. Then it was warnings that were purposely ineffective. Then it was doctors who didn't report adverse reactions. Now it was an entire industry putting money ahead of patient health and lives. It was incredible.

But Alex had quit the prescription drug industry. Maybe he had a bone to pick with them and wasn't being fair. Maybe he was just inclined to the dramatic. One thing I was sure of: if what he said was true, it affected millions of people. And I was sure that most people had no clue it was going on. What surprised me most was the role of the doctors. Why didn't they see how critical it was to read the warnings? Why didn't they take responsibility to report the adverse reactions they saw, to help prevent others?

Big Pharma couldn't claim such low numbers of adverse reactions, unless the people that patients told about them—our doctors—pretended they didn't hear. Health Canada and Big Pharma knew that adverse drug reactions were likely happening a hundred times more often then were ever reported, but they did nothing effective to caution doctors and patients. They both knowingly published numbers of adverse reactions that were a tiny fraction of the truth. The doctors played "Hear No Evil." Any doctors who actually looked at drug labels became victims of collegial indifference, reading prescribing information on drug labels that made the drugs look far less risky than they actually are. It was an unspoken conspiracy of silence. Don't ask. Don't tell.

Clearly marketing blockbusters was the source of the problem. I knew I must follow the money.

SECTION TWO

Follow the Money

Chapter 5

They Knew, and They Didn't Tell

"The cruelest lies are often told in silence."
—Robert Louis Stevenson

April 2000

I SAT AT MY DESK reviewing Alex's stunning insights. Events like Bhopal, India, where in 1984, at least 2,500 people had died due to a chemical gas leak at a Union Carbide plant ran through my mind. More than 1,500 people died when the *Titanic* sank. But these were isolated accidents, where either one person or a small group of decision-makers had made mistakes that ended in a disaster. There was an end date. And "accident" was the keyword. An error. But Alex was talking about corporate plans that end up harming or killing people on an ongoing basis, while omitting to do the things that would protect them. If what Alex said was true, in my view this was corporate crime on a massive level.

I say "if" because I realized I still had some nagging doubts. It went against what I believed about people—that they are basically good. And if I doubted it, who would believe it? Yet if you plan to kill a specific person and they die, it's murder. You go to jail. So why is it that if your plans assume a number of deaths, and you hold back information that could prevent them, it's called good business? If your products also help people; and you contribute to the economy, does that make it okay?

I had worked for fourteen years for Canada's then largest company, Bell Canada. Safety was paramount there. I once attended an awards ceremony for Bell sales reps who'd driven company cars for decades with not one accident—one man thirty-five years. Safety can be managed. How could pharmaceutical companies and doctors that dealt with matters of life and death every day be any less careful? Yet Alex had been an industry insider. He should know. And my conversations with both industry doctors haunted me. I knew I would have to dig deeper. Marketing blockbusters and their side effects made the *Titanic* look like a boating accident.

May 2000

Thank goodness the people I knew in the drug industry were still calling me back. Most of them were very sympathetic but unfortunately gave me little specific information. One afternoon however, I received a call from Jane Cooper. Jane was a veteran Big Pharma insider who'd worked many years for a major pharmaceutical company, but had since left the industry. She was also a parent and friend who was well aware of our loss. I hoped Jane would be as candid with me as Alex Demerse had been.

"The industry people I know are being pretty closed-mouthed," I told Jane.

"That's because the industry code of silence is so powerful," she said. "No one wants to risk losing their job and stock options by talking openly about safety concerns. Even pharma retirees keep quiet. They're all afraid of being sued, and with good cause. They would be."

"The safety warnings the companies send out are confusing," I said.

"The warnings are confusing because the official industry position is that Ottawa deals with safety and efficacy, and it's up to the doctor and pharmacist to supply the information to patients."

I added "Which no one really understands."

"Right," she agreed.

I took a moment to think about that. "Do you mean the drug companies don't accept the responsibility to warn patients about risks and keep them safe when using their drugs?"

"That's right. It's high-level finger-pointing."

To me that was like an auto manufacturer saying it was the dealer's responsibility to warn car buyers about unsafe vehicles.

I asked Jane about blockbusters: "I've been told the industry weighs deaths against billions in sales."

"Of course they do. International CEOs are paid to increase sales. And Big Pharma Canadian affiliates are primarily sales and marketing arms. Canada is small potatoes. The real decisions are made in the U.S. or Europe. Canadian affiliates all kowtow to the head office."

So it might not have been a Canadian that had decided what warnings consumers in Canada would get for Prepulsid, or that Prepulsid would continue to be sold here. Was my search for justice going to take me to the U.S. or Europe?

"I'm considering a lawsuit," I confided. "But I'm not sure where to start."

"You'll have to sue in Canada, but you'll probably be alone. Canadian courts rarely accept class action lawsuits against pharmaceutical companies. And individual lawsuits are rare because adverse drug reactions are very hard to prove. The companies will just blame the doctors. They just won't bend."

Jane was warning me we would probably lose a legal battle.

"I have to do this," I said. "I'm working to get an inquest. What would you do if you were me?"

Jane seemed pleased that I was resolved. "Getting governments to act is very tough. The industry is very well connected to the politicians. They donate to the parties in Canada, and give millions to the party PACs (Political Action Committees) in the U.S. Yet they won't hesitate to sue governments if they cross them. They actually scare governments. You have one chance. They care about two things: sales and share value, and hate the media—especially *60 Minutes* and *20/20*. Call *60 Minutes*. Call CBC. Tell Vanessa's story. Align yourself with U.S. and Canadian advocacy groups. Make sure Vanessa's story doesn't die. It's the only way to get anyone's attention."

Jane had given me a strategy. I knew what I had to do. It was just a matter of how.

And something was troubling me deeply: for how long had the people at Health Canada known the true risks of Prepulsid? Was Vanessa's death just a matter of terrible timing, like a soldier killed minutes after the war was over on Armistice Day?

I was about to find out.

My landlord, lawyer Jeremy Taylor, had prepared a document for Gloria and I that amazed me: "A Brief History of Prepulsid." It outlined the content of the four U.S. "Dear Doctor" Prepulsid warning letters since 1995. I studied it carefully and then did my own research. It turned out that Janssen-Ortho had issued *five different* "Dear Doctor" warning letters about Prepulsid to Canadian doctors on different dates: each time when the official label was changed to add warnings.[1]

Prepulsid had been introduced in Canada in 1989 and

approved in the U.S. in 1993. The official 1989 Canadian Prepulsid label had no warnings related to arrhythmias, long QT, or torsades de pointes.

Within one year the official Canadian Prepulsid label had a new warning: "*Rare cases of serious cardiac arrhythmias, including ventricular arrhythmias and torsades de pointes associated with QT prolongation, have been reported in patients taking PREPULSID (cisapride monohydrate). Some of these patients did not have known cardiac histories; however, most had been receiving multiple other medications and had pre-existing cardiac disease or risk factors for arrhythmias. A causal relationship to Prepulsid has not been established.*"

That was ten years before Vanessa died. Dr. Eggar had characterized the Prepulsid warnings as vague. I could immediately see why. With no causal relationship established who would be concerned? But the label said "most" other patients who suffered arrhythmias had other risk factors. *Most* doesn't mean *all*. Stated differently, that meant that back in 1990, Janssen's own evidence showed that *some* patients on Prepulsid suffered life threatening arrhythmias apparently caused solely by Prepulsid. Why not just say so?

By March 1995 after a number of Prepulsid-related deaths had been reported, Johnson & Johnson changed the prescribing information again to add new safety warnings. And the first of five Canadian "Dear Doctor" letters went out, contraindicating Prepulsid for patients taking the antifungals ketoconazole and itraconazole, for patients who might have long QT, and for those with uncorrected electrolyte disturbances. The letter, signed by Alain Raoult, vice-president of Scientific Affairs at Janssen-Ortho read, "Although a causal relationship has not been established to the above cardiac side effects, we at Janssen feel it prudent to advise you of our product monograph changes."

Once again, no admitted causal relationship. It would

appear the people at Janssen-Ortho were just being prudent. The letter also read, "We have received recent reports of QT prolongation and ventricular arrhythmias, including torsades de pointes in patients taking Prepulsid with other medications, in chronically ill patients and in patients who had other risk factors for arrhythmia." Most doctors would conclude Prepulsid was still quite safe for patients with no other risk factor. But what about the people on Prepulsid mentioned in 1990—who had suffered arrhythmias despite no risk factors? And wasn't it dishonest to imply the reports were only "recent," when arrhythmias had been reported in relation to Prepulsid over five years before?

Later the same year on December 14, 1995, Janssen changed the Canadian label again, and sent out a second "Dear Doctor" letter in Canada, this time contraindicating Prepulsid with fluconazole, and antibiotics erythromycin and clarithromycin, telling doctors "data suggest" that in combination with Prepulsid they might cause long QT. Once again the letter assured doctors that a causal relationship had not been established. "*Worldwide experience indicates that Prepulsid is safe and effective when used in accordance with its labeling,*" the letter stated.

I thought carefully about that. It wasn't true in 1989 because that label mentioned no cardiac warnings. It wasn't true in 1990 because that label didn't mention erythromycin, clarithromycin, or fluconazole (all contraindicated in December 1995).

And it wasn't going to be true in December 1995 either, because in July 1997 Janssen changed the Prepulsid label again, and it had grown from thirty-three to fifty-one pages.

In 1997 Janssen also sent out a third "Dear Healthcare Professional" letter in Canada contraindicating Prepulsid with the antidepressant nefazodone and a group of drugs, protease-inhibitors, as well as use in "*prematurely born infants.*" Significantly, this letter did *not* say "a causal relationship has not been established" but still maintained that "worldwide experience indicates that Prepulsid is safe and effective when used in accordance with its labeling," now proven numerous times to have never been true. Unless "safe" means some people on Prepulsid will probably die.

In the meanwhile U.S. doctors had received a four-page "Dear Doctor" letter about Prepulsid along with the strongest warning the FDA mandated for any prescription drug:

By June 26, 1998, U.S. reports linked thirty-eight deaths to Prepulsid, and after further negotiations with the FDA, Johnson & Johnson placed a "Black Box Warning" on the U.S. label, and on the package insert that *goes right into patient's hands*. Black box warnings appear right upfront in bold print. Any doctor, pharmacist, or patient that looked at any of these three documents could not miss what the warning said in bold: *Serious cardiac arrhythmias including ventricular tachycardia, ventricular fibrillation, torsades de pointes, and QT prolongation have been reported in patients taking PREPULSID. Some of these events have been fatal.*[2]

The U.S. letter also said in bold: *QT prolongation, torsades de pointes (sometimes with syncope) cardiac arrest and sudden death have been reported in patients taking Prepulsid without the above mentioned contraindicated drugs.*

The letter detailed more new risk information and added a long list of new Prepulsid risk factors like terfenadine (Seldane) and astemizole (Hismanal), two classes of antiarrhythmic heart drugs, tricyclic antidepressants, tetracyclic antidepressants, and certain antipsychotics, summing up with, "the preceding lists of drugs are not comprehensive." In other words, we're only giving you part of the story.

The letter also identified new side effects and a potential causal connection for reactions reported by patients taking Prepulsid, including confusion, depression, suicide attempts, and hallucinations.

Importantly for me, the 1998 U.S. "Dear Doctor" letter also read under "Precautions": Prepulsid should not be used in patients with "severe hydration, *vomiting* or malnutrition."

That 1998 U.S. black box warning was the one that might have saved Vanessa's life—had any of her doctors seen it. But in 1998 when Johnson & Johnson placed the highest level of alert they had on Prepulsid to U.S. patients, they refused to issue any similar high-level warning for Canadian patients.

When I first read this I admit I was outraged. A drug is a drug. And a person is a person. How could the people at Johnson & Johnson possibly justify not providing the same strong warnings to Canadians as Americans?

And even the 1998 U.S. Prepulsid warning raised more questions than it answered. Was this long list of contraindications compiled by counting injured patients and dead bodies over ten years? Were the people at Johnson & Johnson just on a voyage of dark discovery? And how could Johnson & Johnson continue to sell a drug with so many contraindications to treat non-life threatening conditions?

I could understand using a risky drug to help control a patient's cancer. It might save or extend their life. The risk would be worth the benefit. But heartburn and bloating? This was the unholy power of a blockbuster. Reading the 1998 "Dear Doctor" letter made me realize it's not what Big Pharma tells you that can kill you, it's what they don't.

With further research I discovered that back in Canada, in September 1998, doctors were sent a fourth "Dear Doctor" letter—four pages long—mentioning new contraindications on the label. But there was still no similar black box warning. And Canadian patients did not get any package insert in their hands from Johnson & Johnson.

On June 1, 1999, Johnson & Johnson sent out a third warning letter to U.S. doctors adding two more contraindications:

"Known family history of congenital long QT syndrome" and bradycardia (slow heartbeat). It also said this: "Co-administration of grapefruit juice with cisapride increases the bioavailability of cisapride and concomitant use should be avoided."

TO ME, THIS WAS A GREAT EXAMPLE of the medical-speak that muddies the waters for risky drugs. It says *something*, but you can't be sure what. How many people would know what "co-administration," "bioavailability," and "concomitant" mean? (They mean giving them to patients at the same time; how much drug gets into your blood and system at one time; and using them at the same time.) An effective warning might have said: "WARNING: NEVER mix Prepulsid and grapefruit juice. The combination could result in death."

But if any patient found the Prepulsid label on the Internet, clear statements like that might scare them away from Prepulsid. Marketers hate that.

And even for the doctors who may have read the faxed letter, "should be avoided" is not a term that really grabs your attention like "IS DANGEROUS." You "avoid" the talkative neighbour in the grocery store. Avoid is a word used to advise people, not warn them.

Anyway, Canadian doctors did not get the June 1999 U.S. "Dear Doctor" letter.

On January 24, 2000, Johnson & Johnson issued their fourth letter to U.S. doctors, which expanded the black box warning, saying serious cardiac arrhythmias "have been reported" in patients taking Prepulsid, and directing doctors to conduct a twelve lead EKG test on patients before administering Prepulsid. The letter also listed the official U.S. numbers of reported arrhythmias (more than 270) and deaths (70).

But "have been reported" is still vague. That's like the

police sending out a letter to homeowners saying: Missing jewels, cash, and TVs *have been reported* in houses with broken door locks.

To muddy the waters further, in the same paragraph it reads:

"In approximately 85 per cent of these cases the events occurred when Prepulsid was used in patients with known risk factors. In approximately 0.7 per cent of these cases, the events occurred in the absence of identified risk factors: in the remaining cases, risk factor status was unknown."

This isn't even medical-speak. It's bafflegab, reminiscent of the classic from U.S. Secretary of Defense Donald Rumsfeld: "There are known knowns. There are things we know we know. We also know there are known unknowns. That is to say we know there are some things we do not know. But there are also unknown unknowns, the ones we don't know we don't know."[3]

It remains unbelievable to me that no one at Janssen, at the FDA or Health Canada had ever put their foot down and said, "This must stop. From now on these warnings will be written so doctors and patients can understand them."

Here's a different way they could have stated the risk factor information:

"For all the heart arrhythmias officially recorded related to Prepulsid since it came on the market, we at Janssen feel it prudent to advise you that by the evidence 15 per cent were apparently caused by Prepulsid all by itself."

Doesn't that sound different?

The label also said "because the cases were reported voluntarily from a population of unknown size, estimates of adverse events frequency cannot be made." Why not? Since the best available evidence is that 1 per cent or less of adverse reactions are reported, to determine the risk, why not multiply the number of reported heart arrhythmias (270) by 100? That would mean

Prepulsid might have caused 27,000 life threatening heart arrhythmias—which should have been enough to pull Prepulsid off the market in January 1999. And since 85 per cent of those—22,950—would probably be due to known risk factors, it was obvious that doctors in the U.S. were not reading the warnings.

If U.S. doctors weren't reading the warnings, what difference would a black box warning make? Big Pharma marketers know that the best place to hide something is in plain view.

At least the fourth "Dear Doctor" provided one saving grace for Prepulsid patients—it demanded action. It directed the doctors to conduct an ECG test on patients before prescribing Prepulsid. Many doctors would quickly conclude that this drug is just too risky for patients if a heart test is necessary. Goodbye blockbuster.

When Prepulsid's blockbuster status finally ended with withdrawal on March 23, 2000, in the U.S. the withdrawal announcement read: "Prepulsid remains safe and effective for the vast majority of patients when used according to the approved prescribing information." Technically, for the vast majority that was true, but cold comfort. They could have added: "...but can be dangerous with a long and growing list of contraindications that continues to surprise us at Johnson & Johnson." They knew that. But they didn't tell.

In Canada, when the fifth and final warning letter was issued to doctors it was dated February 2000 (no day). Canadian patients never got anything like a special black box warning. Janssen added the number of reported arrhythmias (22) and deaths in Canada (6) to the total. But I was amazed to see that even after all the deaths and four previous letters that appeared to do little to reduce injuries and deaths, Janssen-Ortho was still fiddling with the small print to keep sales up. The Canadian letter only directed doctors to conduct the potentially life-saving ECG test on patients suspected of having risk factors for cardiac arrhythmia. This letter ended with "Prepulsid remains safe and effective when used in accordance with its labeling." With five label changes this had never been true. After studying the Johnson & Johnson warning letters closely I knew I had been introduced to the fine art of confusion—otherwise known as Big Pharma linguistics.

In April Jeremy Taylor had taken a drive one day to Buffalo, New York, and dropped into a pharmacy, where he got a copy of the *U.S. Prepulsid Medication Guide*—the information sheet that was given to U.S. patients with their pills—the one no one in Canada got. Here are some key sections starting at the top:

What is the Most Important Information I Should Know About Prepulsid (cisapride)?

PREPULSID may cause serious irregular heartbeats that may cause death.

If you feel faint, become dizzy or have irregular heartbeats while using PREPULSID, stop taking PREPULSID and get medical help right away.

Also, you should not take PREPULSID if you have any of these conditions [the list of nine conditions included]:

• low blood levels of potassium, calcium or magnesium
• an eating disorder (such as bulimia and anorexia)
• your body has suddenly lost a lot of water
• persistent vomiting
The safety and effectiveness of PREPULSID in children younger than 16 years has not been demonstrated for any use. Serious adverse events, including death, have been reported in infants and children while being treated with PREPULSID, although there is no clear evidence that PREPULSID caused them.

I would call that a clearly worded warning. But it was the warning no Canadian patient ever saw. There it was, upfront in bold letters—the consequences that might occur if you had an adverse drug reactions to Prepulsid—"death." That's what had been missing from every warning I'd seen to date—consequences. Consequences hurt sales.

How many parents would allow family members to take any drug that "may cause death"? Certainly not Gloria and I.

Two years later I visited the University of Toronto School of Pharmacy library on Russell Street to research drug names and side effects. I took the elevator to the fourth floor and found myself standing amongst texts on pharmacology. A few students sat quietly reading as I wandered the stacks looking at the titles of manuals. After an hour I found myself staring in awe at the entry for Prepulsid (cisapride) in a thick volume entitled *Drug Interaction Facts*. There were *ninety-nine* entries of drugs, foods or classes of drugs that could interact with Prepulsid. Ninety-one of them were marked as serious. No other drug had a list anywhere near that long. The potentially life-saving antibiotic clarithromycin only had seventeen serious entries—one of them Prepulsid.[4] By August 2007 the website Drug.com listed 525 individual drugs that could cause significant interactions with Prepulsid, still selling in many countries, under many names.

Chapter 6

All Drugs Cause Adverse Effects

"One of the first duties of the Physician is to educate the masses not to take medicine."
—Sir William Osler, Canadian physician (1849–1919)

FOLLOWING JANE COOPER'S ADVICE, in late April I contacted Dr. Sidney Wolfe at Public Citizen in Washington D.C., a not-for-profit public watchdog organization co-founded by Sidney and Ralph Nader in 1961.[1] Public Citizen uses legal action to help ensure the U.S. FDA protects American patients. Sidney heads up their Health Research Group and co-wrote the drug manual *Worst Pills–Best Pills* which helps fund their work.[2] I was told that Big Pharma hate these guys, who are a constant thorn in their side, so naturally I wanted to speak with them. Public Citizen was on top of Prepulsid and had just called publicly for the FDA to order it off the shelves immediately, instead of allowing Johnson & Johnson to keep selling it for four more months until August 17.

Sidney was very helpful. He estimated that as many as twelve people with no other drugs or conditions might have died related to taking cisapride (Prepulsid). He also verified that it would be critical in our case for the forensic exam to find cisapride in Vanessa's blood.

"Cisapride should not be on the market," he said. "They [Johnson & Johnson] changed the labeling five times and still had problems and deaths. And the warnings patients get in pharmacies are useless." He recommended the U.S. Medguide warning I'd seen. "No Canadian warning that we've found to date says any such thing," he told me.

"If only I had heard this before," I thought. The enormity of our loss was never far. Sometimes my head or chest would actually hurt during these conversations while thinking "if only." Like "if only" Health Canada had issued truly effective warnings.

Jeremy Taylor's report also held a buried treasure I thought would increase our chances of winning a lawsuit. It was the minutes from a Health Canada committee meeting fifteen months prior: the Expert Advisory Committee on Pharmacovigilance meeting on November 30, 1998. This is medical-speak for a meeting of Health Canada staff and expert doctors to discuss what prescription drugs might be dangerous. Prepulsid had been under review that day, and, according to the minutes, the experts had very serious concerns about it. "This drug is widely used" and "appears to enjoy much off-label use," the minutes read. "A large number of people will be administered the drug, exposing them unnecessarily to its adverse drug reactions."

So Health Canada officials had openly discussed the dangers as far back as November 1998.

This review had taken place five months after the third Canadian "Dear Doctor" letter had gone out in June. The minutes indicated: the warnings "were not very effective, especially when the manufacturer is the source," and "should have been stated up front in a concise manner." The committee felt the letters were "largely ignored and had little impact."

They had recommended that "an alternate mechanism for disseminating important information about the safe use of drugs should be sought," and discussed different wording for the public and "specially marked brightly coloured envelopes to indicate the source and make it stand out."

These were sound conclusions and good ideas, and the experts concluded, "It has now become a very onerous task for the physician to determine whether the benefits outweigh the risks." That said it all: doctors themselves didn't know if Prepulsid was safe. And minutes are not a full transcript. I wondered what they might have left out.

The minutes exposed a cry for help from the experts for Health Canada to protect patients from Prepulsid. So, what did Health Canada do about it? The next day Jeremy Taylor wrote to the official who had prepared the minutes to ask what actions had been taken. The answer would tell Gloria and me if we had to sue our own government to prevent similar deaths. Those meeting minutes were a revelation in my quest.

"You should consider suing Health Canada along with Johnson & Johnson," Jeremy advised me, "and the doctors who knew Vanessa had been taking Prepulsid, and the pharmacy that had sold you the pills with no warning. But when you sue the government of Canada you must file your suit within six months."

I protested. "But it will take me longer than that to find out what really happened. Why in six months?"

He shrugged. "Because they are the government and they write the rules. That's why."

I had until September 19, 2000, to file a legal claim for damages—less than five months away. This decision would be

painful and fraught with risk. Being up against Johnson &
Johnson would be difficult enough. They were one of the world's
top one hundred companies—worth over $100 billion, and
prescription drugs were a large part of their business. But taking
on the Government of Canada at the same time was daunting.
Health Canada also had virtually unlimited resources for
lawyers—taxpayer's money. Our money. A trial would be
extremely difficult for our family emotionally. The opposition
would know that. I didn't know if we could afford the financial
risk. It could mean spending our life savings, or selling our
home, or both. And what if after many months of litigation
something went wrong and we lost? I couldn't imagine how that
would affect my family. Madeline and Hart were both heading
for post-secondary schools. Could I explain to them we couldn't
help them out financially because I had to keep an oath I'd made
to myself the day after Vanessa died? Gloria and I would need
time to consider all this. I agonized over this decision. There had
to be a way.

I'd been reading a lot about other risky drugs that had been
pulled off the market, and needed to find out how Prepulsid
stacked up against them. The diabetes drug Rezulin had been
pulled off the U.S. market two days after Vanessa died under
similar circumstances, for causing liver damage to patients. A
class action lawsuit was pending over fen-phen, a combination
of diet drugs sold together that had been taken off the market in
September 1997 after being associated with pulmonary hypertension leading to severe heart and lung damage.

I called Larry Sasich at Public Citizen in Washington, Sidney
Wolfe's co-author of *Worst Pills–Best Pills*. He'd heard Vanessa's
story from his fiancé Sana Sukkari, a hospital pharmacist at
Joseph Brant Hospital in nearby Burlington, Ontario. For drug
safety information, I had hit the motherlode. Larry was extremely
helpful, cheerful, and he had an almost encyclopedic memory for

drug names—both generic and brand names—and their side effects. I sat at my desk with a pad in front of me and pen in my hand for my first formal lesson on adverse drug reactions.

"All drugs cause adverse effects," he said frankly. "There is no such thing as a totally safe drug. Adverse reactions are guaranteed to show up with all new drugs. But there are risks that are acceptable, and risks that aren't. We caution patients about risks that aren't acceptable. The decision to take a drug should always be: does the potential benefit outweigh the potential risk."

"I always thought adverse reactions were extremely rare."

"Not really," he said. "A dangerous adverse reaction can happen to virtually anyone. And they happen all the time. If the U.S. government kept track, adverse drug reactions would be the fourth leading cause of death in this country. A study by three Canadians showed there are over 100,000 deaths a year in the U.S. due to drug reactions in hospitals when the drugs are taken *as prescribed*.[3] Outpatient reactions account for many more."

I was astonished. Larry had written the book on drug safety. If this was true, adverse drug reactions were a man-made epidemic. But Larry spoke factually, like Dr. Sidney Wolfe, who knew off the top of his head about the five label changes for Prepulsid. These guys knew everything about Prepulsid that our doctors didn't.

"We knew about the heart arrhythmias for some time," he told me. "And we rated Prepulsid as 'Do Not Use' in our 1999 edition of *Worst Pills–Best Pills*. 'Do Not Use' means we recommend that you don't use it because it's not as safe as the alternatives; or there's a lack of evidence it is effective. Prepulsid has over forty contraindications. One alternative was metoclopramide (Reglan or Maxeran) which is rated for 'Limited Use' itself."

I closed my eyes when I heard Larry's words, as I felt a sharp pain in the front of my head. Just a few weeks too late. A periodic vision had begun to haunt my thoughts. It was Vanessa pouring a Prepulsid pill out of the little plastic bottle into her hand and taking it with a glass of water; then cheerfully heading out to be with her friends. It still haunts me.

"In the previous edition of our book Prepulsid was rated 'Limited Use.'" That was 1994.

Larry explained that "limited use" means published studies state that it should only be used if another drug doesn't work, or if it's less dangerous than another drug. Even back in 1994 Public Citizen had cautioned patients. It didn't surprise me that metoclopramide had a warning for limited use. I remembered that it could cause "oculogyric crisis" from Dr. David Knox.

"Was Prepulsid more effective than metoclopramide?" I asked.

"Maybe for some patients. But not necessarily. With cameras and computers newer is always better, but not drugs. There is nothing that requires a new drug to be any better than an older drug for approval. The companies never compare them to older drugs in head-to-head studies. If they were required to, many new drugs wouldn't be approved."

"So all new drugs cause new side effects, but can be less effective? What kind of medicine is that?"

"It's business," he replied. "In the U.S. Prepulsid is only approved for nighttime dyspepsia [heartburn]. It's approved for gastro-motility disorders in Canada, and the labeling is easier. That leaves the door wide open for prescribing for any gastrointestinal use even if there is no evidence to support safety and efficacy."

So with Prepulsid, Canada had a lower safety standard for new drug approvals and label warnings. Larry also told me that Johnson & Johnson had been caught red-handed breaking the rules—marketing Prepulsid off-label—by the FDA. They had been warned and ordered by the FDA in June 1998 to revise their promotional materials for Prepulsid.

"Why didn't the FDA just order Prepulsid off the market earlier?" I asked.

"The problem is that the relationship between the drug companies and the FDA is a 'service' kind of relationship. A large portion of the FDA drug approval budget comes from fees paid by the drug companies. It's inappropriate for a regulator to be paid by the regulated. They exert too much influence."

I wondered how an FDA drug reviewer would feel ordering a Big Pharma blockbuster off the market when industry money is paying most of his or her salary. And how could reviewers be unbiased in their work? If new drug applications stopped, reviewers would be out of work. Their job security is tied to drug approvals. I later learned that Health Canada is no different, where 60 per cent of the budget for the compliance branch is paid by fees from the industries it is supposed to police.[4] In the film about global warning, *An Inconvenient Truth*, Al Gore quotes Upton Sinclair: "It is difficult to get a man to understand something when his salary depends upon his not understanding it."

I asked Larry if doctors had to report adverse reactions by law in the U.S.

"No. There is no active surveillance system for potential drug injuries. Some European countries have legal requirements to report adverse drug reactions but they are difficult to enforce. We believe the FDA really only gets between 1 per cent to 10 per cent of the true number of serious adverse drug reactions and deaths reported. A lot of doctors never report adverse reactions."[5]

We agreed to speak again, said goodbye, and a minute later my fax machine began to hum. The Public Citizen letter to the FDA started like this: "We have obtained new FDA reports concerning twenty-three additional U.S. deaths since the beginning of this year from cardiac arrhythmias or sudden cardiac arrest/death associated with the use of the heartburn drug, Prepulsid. These are in addition to the eighty previous FDA-announced heart rhythm-associated deaths." It insisted that the FDA take all Prepulsid off the shelves within two weeks "to prevent additional people from being killed by this drug."

Larry and Sidney were certainly on the job. The total Prepulsid associated death toll had apparently risen to 103 deaths. And they hadn't even counted Vanessa and other possible Canadian deaths. What about the other 117 countries Johnson & Johnson sold Prepulsid? What was the real Prepulsid-related death toll?

And something else was troubling me—doctors not reporting adverse drug reactions. I logged onto the Internet and Googled causes of death in the U.S. Larry was right. None of the charts that came up on web pages from various research organizations even mentioned adverse drug reactions as a cause of death. The only thing even close was a catch-all: "unintentional injuries" which included all accidents and all medical errors. The Statistics Canada information appeared the same.

No government was tracking deaths due to adverse drug reactions.

Yet if there were over 100,000 deaths caused by adverse drug reactions in hospitals, they were the *fourth-leading cause of death*—after all cancers, heart disease and strokes. And that didn't include deaths outside hospitals.

Two days later I received a call from Larry Sasich's associate and fiancé, Sana Sukkari, the staff pharmacist at Joseph Brant Hospital in nearby Burlington. She had urgency in her gentle voice. Sana spoke quietly into the phone, as if she was afraid someone would hear her. After offering her sincere condolences about Vanessa, she told me why she called.

"Vanessa shouldn't have had to pay with her life for this drug. I've been aware of the problems with cisapride for some time. I conducted my own study of ten cancer patients given cisapride while in my hospital between 1998 and 2000. One was inconclusive. Of the remaining nine, seven died in our hospital."

I froze, then quickly did some calculations in my head. Seven out of nine is more than 77 per cent—a deplorable record. But people die in intensive care. They were there because they had cancer. That figure itself might not prove anything about Prepulsid.

Sana continued: "In all seven cases where the patient died, cisapride was contraindicated. And in all seven cases the ECG report showed prolonged QT, tachycardia, or cardiac arrest. All of these can be caused by cisapride."

This was a stunning breakthrough. First, seven patients had been given Prepulsid when the official label warned they shouldn't. Second, all seven patients suffered predictable heart rhythm problems. Third, all seven died. The fact that they died after suffering long QT or arrhythmia could not be a coincidence. To me this verified that Prepulsid with its contraindications might be a predictable killer—seven out of seven—100 per cent.

Sana was almost whispering: "None of the cases in the hospital record showed cisapride as a possible cause of death. The families have a right to know." This was what I'd been looking for. Alex Demerse and others had told me that adverse reaction deaths get blamed on overdoses, contraindications, and existing illness. Here was a perfect example with Prepulsid twenty minutes from our home. I pictured families going through funeral arrangements, reading their sympathy cards and mourning as we did, all without knowing the true cause of death may have been a drug error. Sad.

"Can I get a copy of your report?" I asked, trying to sound somewhat disinterested. The report would be powerful evidence to show to the coroner to help get an inquest, and to Health Canada officials to help get Prepulsid off the market in Canada. Our potential lawsuit was on my mind as well. I thought it would be key evidence at a trial. Maybe even winning evidence.

"Health Canada has had all the information since April 4th. Because of patient confidentiality I can't give it to you." My heart sank. I'd just met a health professional with integrity who truly put patients first. But she had too much integrity to give me her report. I admired her courage. Despite her personal risk, Sana was still more concerned about the patients. However, she was taking on four very powerful organizations Johnson & Johnson, her hospital, the doctors, and Health Canada.

"Sana, this is going to embarrass a lot of people." I cautioned her. "It could get ugly for you."

She didn't flinch. "Terence, I am sworn as a pharmacist to act in the best interest of patients. So I sent it to Health Canada because if they act, it could save patient lives in the future. As a pharmacist I had no choice. I thought you deserved to know the facts." I told Sana why I needed that study and suggested she could black out the names, and then give it to me. Even if nobody at Joseph Brant wanted to investigate what she had discovered, she was still trying her utmost to play by the rules. "It will be revealed in time," she told me.

Sana, like me, believed people are generally good. Sadly, life was about to get a lot tougher for her.

I was doing some more calculations in my head. I guessed there might be six hundred hospitals in Canada. And in the U.S. I guessed ten times that, perhaps six thousand.[6] If seven patients died in each hospital related to Prepulsid, which could mean over 46,000 potential Prepulsid–related deaths across North America that remained hidden. Even one per hospital could be 6,600. On the other hand, the patients at Joseph Brant had been in intensive care with cancer in advanced stages. Their cause of death could have been their illness. That's what their families were told. What was the truth?

My conclusion was simple: find out how they died. I decided to expose these seven deaths and insist on a coroner's inquest into them as well. But I had to do it without blowing Sana's cover. I knew her job and career were in jeopardy. Sana had taken a very big chance sending that report to Health Canada for Vanessa and me. I gave her my word I wouldn't reveal the source. We agreed to talk again soon.

June 1, 2000

The "message waiting" light on my office phone was flashing. I stared at it sitting in silence, reviewing how far I had come in two months. Every time I peeled off one layer, another appeared underneath. The industry people I had interviewed fell into three groups. First, those who worked for Big Pharma and told me very little. Despite my frustration at the time, I understand that. Some of them didn't know very much anyway. And for those who did, their livelihood depended on an industry code of silence.

Next were the people who had left Big Pharma, but were still in business—like Alex Demerse and Jane Cooper. I was very grateful they had spoken to me openly and candidly. They were my angels. I understand that they could not make themselves unemployable and risk being sued by criticizing the drug industry openly. No large company would hire someone who went on the public record criticizing their former employer.

Finally I had heard from another kind of angel—a true whistleblower—Sana Sukkari. The courage Sana showed in contacting me was beautiful to behold. It gave me hope. Vanessa would have admired her.

I checked my voicemail before heading home. The first message was good news from Sana. Health Canada had announced Prepulsid would be withdrawn from the Canadian market as a result of cardiac complications. I found the announcement on the Internet.

It read: Dated May 31, 2000. OTTAWA—Health Canada is warning consumers who are using the drug, PREPULSID® (cisapride), of the possibility of rare, but serious, heart complications, including arrhythmias (irregular heartbeat rhythms) and sudden death.

A CLEAR WARNING. Ten weeks after I had first spoken to Health Canada, they had finally acted. But then came the surprise: Health Canada was going to allow Johnson & Johnson to keep selling Prepulsid until August 7, 2000—another sixty-eight days. They'd made this concession, despite this statement in their own announcement: "In most cases, alternative therapies are available." There was no good reason that I could see not to withdraw Prepulsid immediately. By this time I figured I knew Johnson & Johnson's motives. But I tried to imagine what kind of tortured thinking at Health Canada could have led them to such a foolish decision. Until now I had thought of them as the gang that couldn't shoot straight. I was beginning to suspect something more ominous.

My second telephone message was a familiar voice on the other end of the line, my former colleague Elizabeth Witmer, the Minister of Health for Ontario at the time, calling from her car. On a scale of one to ten for integrity, Elizabeth had always been a ten. "Terence, I wanted you to know the Ontario Cabinet had just issued an order to take Prepulsid off the provincial formularies immediately."

This was big.

It meant that the province would no longer pay for Prepulsid for seniors and those on social assistance. Since private drug plans usually followed the province's lead, they would probably do the same. This would be the effective end to the large-scale sale of Prepulsid in Ontario. I had an immediate flashback to the darkest time of our lives—Vanessa's funeral. Elizabeth had sat in a pew with some of our other former caucus colleagues at St. Jude's who had joined us to say goodbye. Former MPP colleagues Frank Klees and Canon Derwyn Shea read the lessons beautifully. It was overwhelming—all these powerful people gathered in Oakville grieving for a fifteen-year-old girl. Had they known the true risks of Prepulsid even a week before they could have acted. And if the people at Health Canada and Johnson & Johnson had been sitting in one of those pews maybe they would have felt the importance of improving our drug regulatory system—and taking Prepulsid off the shelves immediately. So more funerals weren't needed.

Chapter 7

"Sleeping on the Yellow Line"

*"All substances are poisons. There is none which is not a poison.
The right dose differentiates a poison from a remedy."*
—Paracelsus (1493–1541 AD)

"Any drug without toxic side effects is not a drug at all."
—Eli Lilly, Founder of Eli Lilly and Company, one of the world's
largest pharmaceutical companies.

AS THE SCHOOL YEAR WAS ENDING Madeline was preparing to
go to Queen's University in Kingston—three hours away—to
study music. She had not only completed her school year, but
maintained good marks, an amazing feat under the circumstances. Naturally Gloria and I wished she would stay closer to
home, but she had friends at Queen's and we hoped the change
would be good for her. Hart was finishing grade eight and planning to attend the same high school Vanessa had—Oakville
Trafalgar. He had good friends that helped sustain him in those

days. Gloria was still working at St. Peter's Hospital Foundation. The people at St. Peter's had been very kind to her but her fundraising position there required her to visit donors where they worked, including funeral homes, a disturbing reminder of our personal tragedy.

My consultancy was getting busier, and I had to fit in my phone calls and meetings about Prepulsid between client work. I had also been appointed to a part-time position on the board of the Alcohol and Gaming Commission of Ontario. That meant attending monthly board meetings and adjudicating public hearings on liquor and gambling licences in southern Ontario. I continued my research into the history of Prepulsid and other drugs that had been pulled off the market, in the evenings and on weekends.

On June 14, 2000 I received a call that would change our lives. Dr. David Eden had called an inquest into Vanessa's death in Hamilton, perhaps as soon as the fall. Vanessa would have her day in court. I said a silent prayer of thanks. I was incredibly relieved. Finally, some answers, I thought. But I was also profoundly worried, about the process and possible results. Vanessa would lose her privacy at the inquest, something neither Gloria or I felt good about. Her personal life would be under close scrutiny. The forces on the other side were not about to knuckle under, take the blame, and say sorry. And we still didn't have a lawyer.

So I knew I had to make a decision when Jeremy Taylor came into my office to propose a deal. He wanted to help represent us in court in a class action suit against Prepulsid in Canada. Vanessa would be the lead or "representative" plaintiff. He would work with a highly experienced trial lawyer in Toronto—Gary Will. I considered it a blessing that any lawyer would consider taking our case because class actions involving prescription drugs were uncharted territory in Canada in 2000.

And plaintiffs in class actions do not have to pay the lawyers upfront. They work on contingency—getting paid out of any eventual settlement or award made to all the claimants.

I had used up my MPP severance pay and even cashed in some RRSPs in recent months to pay monthly bills, so contingency payment was the only realistic way we could move forward. If we went to trial on our own, something I wanted, legal fees would cost in the hundreds of thousands of dollars.

Jeremy knew I had been receiving calls from other victims, and proposed a financial agreement whereby, amongst other things, I would maintain contact with the victims, invite them into the class action, and continue my research. He would provide office space at no cost and some clerical support. Gloria and I discussed the offer. Jeremy had been a good friend to us. He'd set me up in an office and investigated Prepulsid of his own initiative. We viewed him as someone who had known Vanessa and would demand justice for her. We trusted him to look out for our family's best interests. So we agreed. The next step was to meet Gary Will.

I had a very good idea what kind of trial lawyer we needed. I just wasn't sure that person actually existed. I felt he or she must only work only for plaintiffs. Having seen a glimpse of the incredible influence Big Pharma has, and been introduced in such a dreadful way to the hidden power of blockbusters, there was no way I'd hire a lawyer for Vanessa who had friends in the drug companies, or might be working for the other side next year. I know this sounds naive, but I wanted someone who would fight for Vanessa because he or she believed in justice in their heart.

Second, I had been warned that a common tactic for some lawyers is to never go to trial. They accept cases against drug companies, then immediately start negotiating how much the settlement will be. How seriously would a Big Pharma company take a lawyer who filed a lawsuit to get a public trial, but who everyone in the profession knew never went to court? In my view it was this kind of legal practice that makes it profitable for Big Pharma to keep risky drugs on the market. The idea of two lawyers sitting down and cutting a quiet deal over Vanessa's death was repulsive to me.

Our best weapon would be public trial which would obtain media coverage. So we needed a lawyer who wasn't afraid to take on three very wealthy and powerful organizations in court. We needed someone who had courage.

Third, the parties we were suing all had virtually unlimited funds for lawyers. Pockets don't get any deeper. All three would stay in to the bitter end. Yet we couldn't pay anywhere near these kinds if fees. I needed a lawyer willing to share in our great risk by agreeing to accept payment on contingency.

In Canada there is little or no legal tradition of huge financial awards by juries for punitive damages against large corporations. In fact in Ontario, outside of class actions, contingency fees were actually illegal until 2000. Canadian law pits companies with more money than many countries against individuals who have little chance of being awarded amounts guaranteed to attract the top lawyers. Nice for Big Pharma. Bad for justice. And bad for patients.

So above all else we needed a winner. Basically, Vanessa needed a hero.

When I met Gary Will I liked him immediately. He is mild-mannered and a good listener; he thoughtfully weighs what he hears before responding. As he spoke I imagined Gary in court and felt a judge or jury would find him easy to listen to—and credible. He had conducted over one hundred trials in his career—for plaintiffs, and had a highly specialized personal injury practice representing individual plaintiffs against large institutions such as insurance companies and other large corporations. As a father of two children Gary would sincerely want to see drug safety improved. He had just won a very important case where he helped an elderly couple and their daughter get a jury award of $1 million in punitive damages against the Pilot Insurance Company, the highest award for punitive damages in the history of Canada. The case had been appealed to the Supreme Court of Canada, and Gary was to argue their position in the coming months. Gary fit the bill. With Gary Will I felt we had a chance at getting justice for Vanessa. How my agreement with Jeremy would work with Gary was to be determined, something I assumed would be worked out later.

The good news was that Gary was prepared to represent Vanessa. We had our trial lawyer.

Then we reviewed the bad news. And there was a lot.

First, nothing would happen until a judge agreed to "certify" our class action, Gary explained, "Class actions were created to save the courts time, and avoid multiple trials where the facts are similar. We'll have to argue before a judge that a significant number of people suffered adverse reactions to Prepulsid taking the drug as prescribed, and that there are a number of common issues which make the class proceeding the preferable procedure. This is far from automatic, because some facts will vary in each case."

"Like what?" I asked.

"Well. Almost every plaintiff will have had a different doctor. In a class action only what the class has in common— the drug—is subject to a finding. In a class action, the doctors would not be held responsible."

I found this quite disturbing. It was clear to me that the doctors didn't read drug labels, or even warning letters. If they didn't have to answer for their actions, how would anything change?

"But how long might the case take?"

Gary paused and raised his eyebrows. I could see he was going to break it to me gently. "It's hard to say. With motions and delays, we could be in litigation for years. And then there's the possibility of appeals. It could end up taking five years—or more."

I tried to imagine living the next five years of my life waiting for some kind of justice for Vanessa. The thought was overwhelming. It was impossible to see that far ahead.

Yet I could see why defendants create delays. They are banking on plaintiffs like us engulfed in grief, and anxious for closure, to give in and settle under better terms for them. Ordinary people often can't afford the costs that occur after a death in the family. Funerals cost thousands of dollars. There is time off work and lost income—sometimes long term. Often there are legal costs. Mounting debts and interest add to the tremendous stress of grief. People break down. That's how Big Pharma settles most of its cases.

We were also up against the Canadian Medical Protection Association, Gary said, the group that insures 95 per cent of our doctors against malpractice. They would provide lawyers for the four doctors that treated Vanessa, and access their war chest of about $2 billion to fight us. My research showed they take virtually every case to the wall, regardless of the medical errors their members made.

Gary Will was a straight shooter and he made sure I understood one additional fact: that even if we won a lawsuit, we might lose. How? Gary explained:

"In Ontario when a young person dies, family members can't claim damages for future lost earnings. Under the Family Law Reform Act the basis for damages is loss of 'guidance, care and companionship.' The key legal precedent is 'To Case'—a fourteen-year-old boy who died in a school accident in Toronto. A jury awarded $100,000 each to his parents and $50,000 to his sister—the highest award ever. But even that award is under appeal by the Toronto school board."[1]

Realistically, if we won, those could be the highest amounts any defendant would be ordered to pay. That might not even cover our legal bills.

Gary also explained that even if a jury ordered the defendants to pay a larger amount, judges were allowed to overturn what the jury had awarded. In fact a judge had knocked down Gary's $1 million jury award for punitive damages in the Pilot Insurance Case to $100,000.

How could one person, or even three judges, overrule a legal decision by a jury of six of your peers? This, I learned, is Canadian justice.

The problem is, of course, that $100,000 or $200,000 is no real deterrent to a large corporation, especially one worth tens of billions of dollars. It's like you or me paying a ten-cent library fine.

And that's how we could lose. Even if we won.

A friend put in context how losing $100,000 would impact a Big Pharma company. He'd attended numerous drug company "performance recognition" trips for top salespeople and described them to me. Everyone was treated like royalty; all expenses paid, open bar, and open buffet all week. One year it was a cruise for three hundred to the French and Italian Riviera—including visits to Nice, Monte Carlo, and San Tropez. In another they booked the entire Four Seasons Resort on the Caribbean island of Nevis. These events would cost at least ten thousand dollars per person, over $3 million. I was saddened to imagine how comparatively insignificant the cost of Vanessa's death as valued by Ontario courts would be to a Big Pharma company—less than a day in the sun for the top sales reps.

Yet in the U.S. potential damages could be in the millions—which attracts some of the best lawyers with contingency fees, and at least stands a chance of improving corporate risk-management practices. If Canadian courts don't value Canadian lives enough to provide a level field, why would international companies value them either? Under international risk management practice, compared to the U.S., causing the death of a Canadian would be a bargain. That's the main reason Canadians don't get effective safety warnings such as black box warnings on risky prescription drugs. And that's why significant damages being awarded to victims in courts are so important.

Gary had done his own research. "Vanessa's case is drawing interest from lawyers across North America," Gary said. "Because it was a 'clean' death related to Prepulsid—something that's been hard to find.[2] Your inquest will be the first out of the chute in North America."

"What does that mean?" I asked.

"It's legal jargon meaning your case will be the first case to come before a jury—and the media. Hundreds of plaintiffs have filed Prepulsid lawsuits across the U.S.[3] Their lawyers want to see how a jury decides the facts about Prepulsid."

I'd seen the websites for U.S. lawyers willing to take on Prepulsid cases all over the Internet. Even though this would only be an inquest where no fault is decided, lawyers on both sides of the issue wanted to see if a jury would find that Prepulsid caused Vanessa's death—a "clean" death. If they did, it would be an indicator that other juries in civil trials might do the same. The stakes were huge. It wasn't just reputation for the doctors or the government. For a company the size of Johnson & Johnson it meant hundreds of millions of dollars in potential court-ordered damages or settlements, and possibly worldwide withdrawal of Prepulsid. That could also slash their revenues share value. This was not good for us. It meant that our opponents would bring all their resources to bear at the inquest.

What I didn't know then was how far they would go.

Jeremy Taylor brought in a very bright high school co-op

student and we began in earnest to gather every bit of information we could about Prepulsid. And there was a lot. Prepulsid had a sketchy history even before it was approved in Canada. I also began setting up meetings with Prepulsid victims for Jeremy and me. There was no shortage of them either. By 2002 there were hundreds of potential class action members in Canada involved in trying to certify a class action lawsuit here. And that was before the class action could even be advertised, because it was not yet certified.

By June I had begun to see some small signs of progress. Larry Sasich called from Washington to tell me some countries in Europe had stopped the sales of Prepulsid—temporarily suspending the Prepulsid product license while reviewing its benefit–risk ratio. But Johnson & Johnson had not voluntarily withdrawn Prepulsid in Europe. I guessed they felt the Europeans should figure things out for themselves, just like Canadians. They had shareholders to answer to.

Sana called in late June. Health Canada still had not released her report, so I couldn't talk about it openly. But she'd been taking some heat about her patient advocacy at work. She was quite nervous, and afraid of losing her job. One afternoon she found a rubber glove with a finger cut off on her desk—a not-so-subtle intimidation.[4] I introduced her to lawyer Jeremy Taylor, with the hope he could help get her situation at work improved, which he did.

I was still leading a double life. I had new clients and was getting results for them during the day. At night I'd sit in front of my computer screen like a ghost, mesmerized, Googling drug names or scientific terms I often didn't understand.

But it was good to be busy. All of us in the family were taking one day at a time. Madeline and Hart spent most of their time with friends. And Gloria was busy with work and managing the house. I admit I wasn't as available to all of them as I should have been. But frankly, we were all like the walking wounded. There were times when none of us could think of anything to say about what was on our mind the most—Vanessa. Being busy with others outside the family actually helped.

My research began to turn up scientific evidence. I'd begun to connect with many scientists and researchers on the Internet. If I found a research paper that showed the risks of Prepulsid, I'd email the researcher who wrote it. I discovered I could get the email address of virtually any professor in the world on university websites. No matter how busy they were, most would reply within a few days. I studied every drug I could find that could cause long QT. Most, like Prepulsid and erythromycin, were contraindicated for each other. Then one night I typed in "cisapride" and "long QT," hit enter and a Google headline appeared: "Effects of cisapride on QT interval in children." Jackpot.

The study had been completed at the Department of Pediatrics at Children's Hospital Los Angeles, and published in the *Journal of Pediatrics* in July 1998. The researchers had performed an ECG test on 101 children on cisapride. All 101 of the children's hearts were affected. The researcher's conclusions: "Cisapride significantly lengthened the QT with a mean increase of 15.5 milliseconds. We conclude that cisapride use is associated with a modest increase in QT interval." What did this medical-speak mean? How important could 15.5 milliseconds be? I dug deeper and the answer sickened me.

The average QT interval in men's hearts is 420 milliseconds—less than half a second. But for women it is 440 milliseconds—twenty thousandths of a second more. Experts say a QT interval of 450 milliseconds significantly increases the risk of arrhythmia. So female patients were more likely to experience a heart arrhythmia, even before they took cisapride. The 15.5 milliseconds added by Prepulsid might push them over the top to 455.5—into the danger zone.

Prepulsid could cause long QT and arrhythmia on its own. It was never approved for children. It was contraindicated with persistent vomiting. Being female was a fourth reason Vanessa should not have been given Prepulsid.

Anne Rochon Ford helped me understanding this issue. She was co-founder of Women and Health Protection, an advocacy group that evolved out of DES Action. The prescription drug DES (diethylstilbestrol) had been marketed to women to prevent miscarriage in the 1950s, but in some cases caused permanent damage to the reproductive organs of their offspring—vaginal cancer in girls and testicular cancer in boys. The members of DES Action were the daughters of DES patients—and victims of DES.

In the early stages of my journey I began find a lot of highly dedicated women involved in prescription drug safety, and asked Anne why.

"One reason is that women have been harmed more by prescription drugs," she said, "They have more adverse drug reactions."

This was new to me. "Why?"

"Because women take more drugs. Women are socialized to be more open about social problems, so for example, more women see doctors about depression and end up on antidepressants. And they are the targets of marketing efforts because they have more exposure to the healthcare system as gatekeepers of health care in the home. More women take care of children and aging parents. Check the ads in any women's magazine."

"So it's primarily the number of drugs taken?"

"No. Women's hormonal makeup is also different, and our biology is more complex: We have babies. We menstruate. We have menopause. Yet women aren't included in most drug trials because they might be pregnant or become pregnant. Drugs are approved based on research on men. Adverse reactions that might only affect women don't appear until the drug is sold on the open market. By that time thousands of women are taking it."

That made sense to me. I'd also read that women have less androgen, a male hormone that may decrease sensitivity to some drugs.

"I've read that women have longer QT, raising the risk of heart arrhythmia."

"Women do have longer QT. That plays out in other drugs as well. But the fact that there's a sex difference for the QT interval is not generally well-known. Drugs are approved too soon, and accepted on faith. Sometimes women pay the price."

In 1998 Johnson & Johnson had been scrutinizing Prepulsid closely. They'd already sent out three warning letters to Canadian doctors, and the last one in October 1997 had contraindicated Prepulsid for premature infants. Surely their scientists would have seen the cisapride ECG study on children in the July 1998 issue of the *Journal of Pediatrics*. And they must also have known the special risk for females. Why didn't they issue a specific warning for children and female patients at that time— especially for those like Vanessa who were *both*?

Surely the people in the drug industry know that secrecy can kill.

There was more on the Internet. A lot more. The World Health Organization had issued a warning that cisapride could cause heart rhythm disturbances *in a repeated way*. This is the gold standard of adverse reactions, leaving no doubt. I printed every relevant study and saved them in a binder for Gary Will. I knew the day was coming when they would be crucial to proving our case.

In late June, Jane Cooper called out of the blue. She still had contacts in the drug industry and told me something that boosted my resolve: "I'm hearing some good things out of Health Canada. The drug companies have felt repercussions. They've

sharpened up, because they know people like you will stand up."
I hadn't seen any changes, but if the Big Pharma companies had
made any improvement behind the scenes I was pleased.

More good news was that Vanessa's story had taken root.
The media were coming to me. I received a call from a documentary filmmaker, Erna Buffie. Erna and her producer Elise
Swerhone wanted to tell Vanessa's story on film for television,
with me on camera. This could be a godsend. A film would be
a televised alert. There were hundreds of thousands of people
out there taking prescription drugs under unsafe conditions.

But media interviews were one thing, a film was another.
Would it be fair to my family to tell Vanessa's story on national
television? My quest had become my way of grieving for our
loss. It was my fuel—allowing me to try to get something positive out of our tragedy. To fill the empty space. And I knew in
my heart that Vanessa would approve. But people grieve differently. Our lives had been turned upside down. Everyone at home
was striving so hard for some normalcy. I wanted to ensure that
my family supported the idea. Erna was going to tell the world
about Prepulsid anyway. Did I have to be the front man?

Erna had done considerable research, and recommended I
talk to Dr. Ray Woosley at Georgetown University. He was a
leading authority on long QT and knew a lot about Prepulsid. In
a tragic coincidence, Ray's own brother had died after taking it.
I agreed to get back to Erna in the coming weeks about her film.

Clearly I had to learn more about adverse reactions. If
prescription drugs caused one hundred thousand U.S. deaths in
U.S. hospitals every year, and many more outside hospitals why
did so few people know? It was mind-boggling. On one hand I
had some highly credible, top-notch professionals like Larry
Sasich who were clearly and calmly explaining how the drug
safety system had been undermined. I felt like they were saying,
"So, you learned the drug industry's dirty little secret the hard way."

On the other was Vanessa's doctors, the government of Canada, the U.S. government and some of the world's largest companies, whose position was, "These things can happen. Trust us."

Late in July my mother and best friends Rik and Jeanette Emmett—Vanessa's godparents—had separately suggested Gloria and I take Madeline and Hart on vacation. When I demurred they both asked if they could help pay for the trip. That's how wonderful good friends and family were to us during that difficult time. I accepted and we drove to Sanibel Island, Florida, a tiny island covered with palm trees—a tropical village. Madeline's longtime friend Alyse joined us. I suppose it was not the best choice for us, because we'd been there with Vanessa two years before and everything reminded us of her. But I had leased a new van, and driving down made the trip affordable.

It had been five months since we lost Vanessa, but life was still quite surreal. Grief came in waves. Sometimes one of Vanessa's favourite songs would come on the Windstar radio and I would pull up at the next traffic light trying to hide my tears. I never before noticed how many television shows and movies have dramatic scenes showing someone desperately trying to revive a loved one. Only they all succeeded, where I had failed.

One afternoon as I sat in Sanibel's warm shallow waves a small fishing hook in the sand pierced my finger. I drove to a small drugstore to get some ointment. As I waited, I watched the elderly pharmacist give a prescription drug to another customer. He patiently explained to the lady how to take her medication, what the side effects might be, and cautioned her what not to take it with. This was a far cry from what I'd experienced at home, which was being handed a computer printed sheet of paper along with my pills as I paid.

I struck up a conversation with him. Michael Green was a retired drug researcher. I asked him about grapefruit juice, which is abundant in Florida. He took a roll of bright orange stickers out of a drawer: Do not take with grapefruit juice.

He said he ordered them to be printed himself. He checked every drug that was contraindicated for grapefruit juice, warned the patient, and personally placed one of these stickers on the patient's bottle of pills.

I was struck with the irony. Here I was in a village on a tiny island where a semi-retired pharmacist had initiated on his own what some of the world's wealthiest companies and most powerful regulators refused to do to save human lives. He also told me he refused to fill prescriptions for doctors he called "writers"—the doctors who write too many prescriptions for Valium and similar drugs. His concern was that the patients were getting far too much. And he provided a written warning with all prescriptions and asked the patients to sign that they received the pills. This was truly "informed consent," like patients provide for non-emergency surgery. For me, this elderly gentleman in his little island shop had a higher safety standard than Big Pharma, the FDA and Health Canada.

That evening I was reading a thriller I'd picked off the shelf in our apartment. In it there was a reference to a macho daredevil who would get drunk and fall asleep on the solid yellow line on a highway to show how fearless he was, totally ignoring the cars and trucks whizzing by in the darkness. If any of the cars drifted across the yellow line he'd be injured or killed. My mind wandered. Fear still preoccupied me. Taking prescription drugs could be like sleeping on the yellow line. I wondered how many people were asleep in their beds at that moment with no idea they were at risk from a prescription drug they were taking. No one ever warned them they could have an adverse reaction at any time.

I hate it when fear is justified. I didn't know it then, but hundreds of people were being injured by heart attacks and strokes related to Vioxx at that time; as many as 56,000 of them died from 2000 to 2004—the greatest drug "crash" in history. In July 2000, tens of thousands of innocent patients on Vioxx were sleeping on the yellow line and didn't know it.

After returning from Florida, on August 9, 2000 I had my first lesson on statin drugs—the ones that lower so-called bad cholesterol. At the urging of my new friends at Public Citizen, Bayer Corporation had "voluntarily" pulled Baycol (cervistatin) off the market the day before, for causing rhabdomyolysis, a painful condition that causes breakdown of muscle cells and can sometimes lead to fatal kidney failure. Forty people had died worldwide. The withdrawal letter read: "Rhabdomyolysis is a serious, potentially fatal, adverse effect of all statin drugs, including Baycol." In other words, it's not just our drug, check out the other statins. This was the twelfth prescription drug in four years to be pulled off the U.S. market for injuring or killing patients since 1997. By this time I was totally engrossed in the hidden dangers of pharmaceuticals. I was starting to think of them as a plague.

Chapter 8

A Message in a Bottle

"There is no incentive for companies to find problems with safety once a drug is approved. It is just downside risk. We find a drug is unsafe when the bodies accumulate."
—Dennis T. Mangano Ph.D., M.D., Founder, Chief Scientist and CEO, Ischemia Research and Education Foundation, *Forbes Magazine*: May 8, 2006

July 2000

EARLY IN JULY I met my second whistleblower, Michele Brill-Edwards.[1] From 1988–1992 Michele was Health Canada's senior physician in charge of prescription drug approvals. Her job was to supervise the doctors that say "yes" or "no" to letting new drugs on the market. This is a long and tedious process that must done with extreme care to protect human lives. The average new drug application (NDA) arrives at Health Canada as a truckload of boxes. It takes months to go through them. Michele had refused to submit to pressure from senior bureaucrats and industry to approve unsafe drugs. This made her very troublesome to the senior bureaucrats at Health Canada. Michele and others even took Health Canada to Federal Court and won a decision to remove a Health Canada director who was overruling sound drug safety decisions. This win cost her the senior position and Michele resigned in 1996.

From that time forward Michele has worked to expose the undue and unseen influence of Big Pharma on our secretive drug approval process. Michele is a doctor who truly put patients first. As soon as I heard about Michele from Larry Sasich, I knew I had to meet her.

We spoke on the telephone and Jeremy Taylor suggested we all go out to dinner. It was a warm July evening when we pulled up at his favourite Mediterranean restaurant, Joso's, a converted old house in Toronto's Yorkville. Michele joined us at a small table on the second floor near the back. After introductions I began to ask Michele some pointed questions. I was hoping she could help me decide if I should include Health Canada in our lawsuit. To win against the government you have to prove a government agency was negligent in carrying out their own policy. That is very difficult, I was warned. They have dozens of staff who take meticulous notes about everything they do and make good witnesses in court.

I knew from Jane Cooper and others that if I was going to change things, the inquest jury would have to decide who had failed to protect Vanessa. I hoped their comments would expose fault. If there was no fault, no foul. My greatest fear was that the inquest jury would become confused and absolve all the parties of any responsibility, like it was just an unfortunate accident.

Luckily we had an ace in the hole. Michael Li was the bureaucrat designated to take the minutes of the November 1998 meeting at Health Canada. He also took meticulous notes, the ones Jeremy Taylor got off the Internet. The expert advisors had told Health Canada officials that the previous "Dear Doctor" warning letters about Prepulsid were "largely ignored and had little impact," and recommended they find a new way to warn doctors about the safe use of drugs. A key suggestion was to mail out warnings in "specially marked brightly coloured envelopes to indicate the source and make it stand out." Had Health Canada followed up and done so with Prepulsid?

Had they directed Janssen to do so?

From my years in business I knew there were many direct mail companies from Montreal to Toronto that would have gladly done the job in a few weeks. Just think of the attention-grabbing mail you get to sell you things like long-distance services and cars—brightly coloured envelopes in different shapes, with catchy phrases to entice you to open them. All the direct mail companies would need is the mailing list of doctors and the text of the warning, and they could mail out a standardized warning to doctors almost guaranteed to get their attention. It could announce in large bold red letters:

Warning for Doctors about Prepulsid.
Important safety information enclosed.
Read immediately.

Of course there were other things Health Canada could have done in 1998 to help protect patients on Prepulsid—like placing notices in the newspapers, calling a press conference, limiting Prepulsid availability to special access only—or withdrawing its license.

Michael Li had written back to Jeremy the day before our meeting with Michele, telling him what actions Health Canada had taken to warn doctors about Prepulsid since that November 1998 meeting. His reply?

The *Canadian Medical Association Journal* has a quarterly insert called the "Canadian Adverse Drug Reaction Newsletter."

An article was placed there in January 2000—fourteen months later. That's it. That's all they did.

Michele was candid about what goes on behind the scenes at Health Canada. Jeremy and I sat surrounded by Joso's colourful décor and ate sea bass and crème caramel while she held us spellbound. I learned more about how bureaucracy really works from Michele that evening than I did in four years as MPP at Queen's Park. I told her about Health Canada's article in the "Adverse Drug Reaction Newsletter."

"They put a message in a bottle," she told me bluntly. Despite all that Michele had been through, she always remained composed and professional. I never sensed any bitterness in her.

"They know most doctors don't read it."

"What about a warning for Prepulsid?" I asked.

"Drugs are dangerous products that must be very carefully regulated. Prepulsid should have been a last-resort drug. It wasn't. They had a duty to order the issuance of a "Dear Doctor" letter within forty-eight hours saying 'This is life-threatening,' and have the final say on the text of that letter."

When I heard this, I was wondering how I would tell Gloria. That was the moment I felt in my heart that the government of Canada was partially to blame for Vanessa's death—through inaction. Health Canada had been given expert advice on what to do to warn doctors and protect patients, and totally ignored the advice. I later checked the article they wrote for that newsletter, published two months before Vanessa died.[2] It contained no directions for doctors whatsoever, and omitted the most important information: the eighty associated deaths in the U.S.—as if Prepulsid was only sold in Canada. In fact it carefully accounted for twelve reported deaths in Canada—blaming all but three on anything except Prepulsid itself.[3] The article read like it was written by the same Johnson & Johnson officials that wrote their "Dear Doctor" letters.[4]

"They negotiated with Johnson & Johnson for weeks over the wording of the "Dear Doctor" letter in January." I replied. "If they had just issued it, I know Vanessa would be alive."

"They shouldn't have negotiated. When life is in danger Health Canada doesn't need to negotiate with anyone. There are precedents. In the late 1980s we acted unilaterally within forty-eight hours at Health Canada with AZT (the AIDS drug). We wrote to the U.S. National Institutes of Health[5] who had been working on AZT to get their research results—because we felt we had a public duty to save lives from AIDS. The NIH people were taken aback, but sent it to us. We approved AZT within forty-eight hours."

"Why didn't they anyone act that quickly with Prepulsid?" I asked.

"The problem is the close association with the pharmaceutical industry, and looking to the interests of the industry rather than the interests of patients."

Here we go again, I thought. Basically what Larry Sasich had said about the FDA.

Michele continued. "The government didn't want to rock the boat since the industry was expanding in Canada," she continued, "Drug companies persuade politicians using carrots—plants, jobs, and political donations—and intimidate them with a stick, thinly veiled threats that the plants will close. They get right to the top: federal fundraising limits don't apply to leadership candidates. They can give as much as they want.[6] The relationship is inappropriate. The Drugs Directorate Laboratory was the Scotland Yard behind the approvals process, questioning products before they were approved. But it was closed in 1997 to save $10 million. Now the Drugs Directorate budget of about $100 million is mostly 'cost recovery,' meaning the pharmaceutical companies pay most of it for approvals, like a customer-client relationship." It seemed like everyone could see the conflicts except the government. Michele was proof: they shot the messenger rather than change the system. And this was the third time I'd heard that Big Pharma intimidates governments—something that alarmed me.

I told Michele that in the U.S. there had been a black box warning for Prepulsid since 1998. And that the revised warning in January 2000 got the attention of many U.S. doctors. "Health Canada should have just copied the FDA warnings in 1998 and January of 2000. Instead they had senior bureaucrats acting in favour of the company, trying to keep the drug on the market. No effective warnings got out in time, and Vanessa died as a result. A decision to not do something is a decision."

I felt totally demoralized. It was called the Health Protection Branch. Where was the protection?

"Why did Health Canada approve a potentially life-threatening drug in the first place, for a non-life-threatening condition?"

Michele smiled regretfully. She knew this was painful for me.

"It's happened before. I had to leave Health Canada because I fought the approval of unsafe drugs and insisted on clear warnings. I fought to prevent approval of Imitrex, a migraine drug that sometimes causes heart attacks and strokes. A dose that's effective for one patient can be three times as much as another patient needs. It has a very narrow therapeutic index (meaning the difference between a helpful dose and a deadly dose isn't very much). Drugs are not one size fits all. Imitrex works by causing restrictions of the blood vessels in the brain. Unfortunately it can also do that to the blood vessels in the heart. It should be marketed in a smaller dose."

"Why would Health Canada approve a dosage that isn't safe?" Jeremy interjected.

"Safe is always relative," she replied.

Michele then described how Big Pharma and our regulators have given a whole new meaning to the word "safe."

"Safe means relative to the condition you are treating and other drugs. In the late eighties the patent protection for Motilium was probably running out so Prepulsid became the new 'safe' drug.[7] The same thing happened with the allergy drug Seldane. It had been also been responsible for a number of deaths due to heart arrhythmia. But it wasn't taken off the market until its manufacturer had Allegra to replace it.[8] So it was 'safe' until there was a new drug to replace it. Then it was 'not safe.'"

I was astounded. The drug companies determine what is "safe" for us based on the next blockbuster they have to sell. Safe doesn't mean without harm. It means less harmful than some other drug!

So up to December 1997 it was okay to take a potentially life-threatening drug—Seldane—for a runny nose. But Hoechst Marion Roussel didn't take it off the market until they had the runny-nose market covered with Allegra. Safe is a shell game. It moves when Big Pharma says it will move, based on what they have to sell, and when they are ready to sell it. I was beginning to realize what is fundamentally wrong with modern medicine. Big Pharma totally dominates our health care. Medicine is all about which drug you should take, instead of "should I take a drug at all"?

Why are Big Pharma sales our regulator's concern? If an automobile manufacturer is selling an unsafe car, a recall is ordered—period. They don't wait until the new model is out, crossing their fingers for no more injuries in the meanwhile, to help the industry.

"If drugs have to be proven 'safe and effective' to get on the market," I asked Michele, "What is the definition of 'effective'?"

"In clinical tests 'effective' means compared to placebo—a sugar pill. A drug can be only slightly more effective than a sugar pill and still get approved. The problem is that doctors assume and believe that new drugs are better than older drugs. They rely on what the industry tells them. But they often aren't."

It was appalling to hear that doctors are that naive. "Why do our regulators even approve drugs that aren't as effective as the ones already on the market?" I asked.

"Commercial rights. The law doesn't require new drugs to be better, because drug companies have a right to make money. The drug companies don't have to compare a new drug in clinical tests to any other drug. Effective does not mean more effective than the drugs already on the market."

"But every new drug has new risks. The least they could do is make sure the risks are for a good reason."

Michele smiled. "I agree."

"Let me get this straight," I summarized. "A drug declared safe and effective by Health Canada might actually be life-threatening to some patients, yet only slightly more effective than water. So there's no way the benefits could outweigh the risks?"

"That's right."

"How often does that happen?"

"It's routine."

"So who is protecting the public?" I asked.

"By statute it is the duty of the Minister of Health through the department to uphold the Food and Drugs Act. The minister is supposed to protect the public from health hazards and fraud in the sale and use of foods, drugs, cosmetics, and medical devices. That is not happening."[9]

"What about the drug companies," I asked. "Don't the risk-management practices help protect the patients?" Michele's reply was an awakening.

"Risk management is not patient protection. Risk management is corporate terminology for making money with responsibility."

A light went on in my head. I had always thought risk management referred to the risk *to the patients*. I remembered what Alex Demerse had told me. "From their view it's better to keep selling it if the lawsuits are minimal—especially in Canada. It's just a cost of doing business." If they start losing in court, he'd said, their insurance will cover most of the costs.

So *that* was risk management. It wasn't the risk to patients they were worried about. It was risk to the corporation! Risk management is a practice that puts human life on the same continuum as money. Money versus lives. Lives versus money.

It turns out risk management was how the auto industry got into such deep trouble in 1965, after startling revelations made by Ralph Nader in his groundbreaking book *Unsafe at Any Speed*. The GM Corvair had a problem—it would roll over at certain speeds. Consumers were outraged when they discovered that the automobile manufacturers had known about safety problems all along but hidden the truth from the public and didn't tell the public. They callously calculated how much any liability would cost the company, assessed the risk, kept selling the cars, and paid out settlements from their profits.

That had been thirty-five years ago. How many people were alive today because of changes in the auto industry—safer designs, seat belts, air bags and recalls? When it came to safety, the auto industry had improved. Big Pharma was still stuck in the sixties,[10] a frightening thought.

How powerful must an industry be to have never been legislated in over forty years to update safety practices that address over one hundred thousand deaths a year in hospitals alone?

I was finding it very hard to understand why I had not heard this incredible story before and asked Michele. "The bureaucrats are there to protect innocent children, seniors, everybody. Yet they support the industry against effective safety warnings. How could anyone work against safety?"

"It's too difficult to believe," she answered. "This is why it's so hard to change things at Health Canada. People find it so scary. They refuse to believe their government is working against them."

We thanked Michele profusely as she got into her cab, and agreed to talk again. Jeremy and I said very little on the drive back to Oakville.

Gloria and I had always taught our children they were incredibly lucky to live in Canada. I recalled a happy time—the first time we listened to Vanessa and her classmates sing "Oh Canada"—her grade one concert at Abbey Lane School. "We stand on guard for thee," the children sang. But shouldn't loyalty work both ways? Wasn't there an unspoken promise for the government to stand on guard for Vanessa? The government and Health Canada had broken faith with the rest of us. And Vanessa paid the ultimate price.

There was no doubt I would sue Health Canada along with the others.

Sometimes as I drove to meetings or worked alone in my office I could hear Vanessa's voice saying "Do it, Dad. Keep going." Yet as I became more determined to expose our faulty drug surveillance system and risks from prescription drugs, my family was trying to recapture some measure of happiness in their day-to-day lives—a far different direction. When I raised the idea of me going on camera for Erna Buffie's film they were not thrilled. I could see why. Our loss was one thing. But my research and advocacy was a constant reminder of the awful circumstances. At home I tried to talk about everything else, but it was getting in the way of my family's healing. They were trying to get used to the fact that life isn't fair. And I was desperately trying to somehow make it so.

One evening I went out to rent a movie to watch at home. Even the movie titles at our video store reminded me of Vanessa, like *Sleeping Beauty* or *Girl, Interrupted*. Most married couples split up after losing a child, in part because parents who've lost a child suffer from guilt; also because people grieve differently. When one spouse needs to talk about the child who has been lost, the other might find that very painful. My own way of dealing with grief was public advocacy. Gloria preferred privacy. So my research and advocacy has put strain on both of us. But she understands why I had to do it. Thank God Gloria and I are still together—now married for twenty-eight years.

Meanwhile our own home was the most potent reminder of this wonderful person who was no longer in our lives. We'd lived there since Vanessa was two years old. I could feel her presence in every room.

Chapter 9

And Man Created Blockbuster

"The quality of mercy is not strain'd, It droppeth as the gentle rain from heaven upon the place beneath."
—William Shakespeare, *The Merchant of Venice*

IN 1943, founder General Robert Wood Johnson established a corporate credo for Johnson & Johnson that still appears on its website:

Our Credo

We believe our first responsibility is to the doctors, nurses and patients, to mothers and fathers and all others who use our products and services . . .

During the rest of August I was busy chairing hearings for the Alcohol and Gaming Commission and working for my clients. Hart was preparing for high school, and Madeline for

Queen's University. In September Madeline was heading off to first year to study music. Her determination and sense of purpose were a source of delight to Gloria and me. A high school friend, Karen, would be her roommate and although she'd never been away from home for more than two weeks, we felt the challenge and fresh start would be a blessing for her. When the day for her departure arrived, Hart joined us as we packed her belongings in our van and drove to Kingston, staying overnight at the Holiday Inn. Madeline's and Hart's inner strength amazed us. Watching them carry on with school and friends as they did struck me as courageous.

The next morning when the residence doors opened, I climbed the stairs to the fourth floor lugging a small refrigerator. Typical of university accommodations, the room built for one had been converted into a room for two with bunk beds. The only place I could fit the refrigerator was on top of a dresser. You couldn't swing a cat. Madeline was right behind me, boxes in hand. The crowded room was totally unexpected, and I was concerned that she would be upset, perhaps even want to leave. I waited to see if we should bother unloading the van. Madeline looked around for a few seconds, then sized up the fridge on the dresser. "It's going to be great," she said.

That was the moment I knew Madeline was going to be fine in Kingston; that despite the huge space in our lives, each of us was moving forward and she would manage what fate had handed us.

We spoke occasionally throughout the fall on the phone. Madeline always cheerfully brought us up to date on her classes and friends, and asked me how work was going. We didn't talk about Vanessa. I couldn't. It was strange: talking about my research and our legal case was fine for me. But talking about our life with Vanessa was physically painful for me. Although my activity was weighing Madeline down, she was considerate enough to not show it.

Michele Brill-Edwards had recommended that I meet with Dr. Neil Shear, who was head of dermatology at Sunnybrook & Women's College Health Sciences Centre in Toronto. Dr. Shear was also the director of the University of Toronto Drug Safety Research Group, and founded the Drug Safety Clinic at Sunnybrook in 1985. He was the founding chair of CADRAC, the Canadian Adverse Drug Reaction Advisory Committee of Health Canada.[1] He was present at the November 1998 meeting when outside experts advised Health Canada officials on Prepulsid.

I called him and he kindly agreed to see me. It was a sunny morning as I drove across Toronto's Highway 401 and down Bayview Avenue, turned into the big Sunnybrook hospital campus, and pulled into the underground parking garage. Neil's office was in one of a maze of older buildings with long hallways covered with institutional-green paint. It looked like a researcher's office from a Hollywood movie set. He sat amidst towering stacks of books, reports, and files that covered his desk and tables. In a frank and cheerful manner Neil educated me on adverse effects, Prepulsid, and the drug industry.

"The large pharmaceutical companies are research-based, but financially driven." he explained. "The clinical studies they publish are chosen by the marketers, based on what will help sales, as opposed to scientific value." In other words, as Alex Demerse had explained to me, the marketers pay for studies that will help sales.

"Does Prepulsid cause long QT?" I asked.

"Yes, it does. It looks like people knew cisapride was dangerous. It was a complicated drug to use safely—unmanageable. We took Prepulsid off our formulary [out of the hospital] over a year ago."

It was painful to hear this. If Dr. Neil Shear worked at our Oakville Hospital I suspected Dr. Kayner would have heard about the risks related to Prepulsid.

By "people" I assume Neil meant people in the industry and researchers. Johnson & Johnson would have known that the professionals at some hospitals had ordered Prepulsid out a year before. They track sales in every hospital closely through IMS Health,[2] I had also spoken to Dr. Alan Kaplan[3] at the Toronto General Hospital, who told me they had also stopped using Prepulsid in his clinic a year before.

"Since all drugs cause side effects," Neil explained, "there will always be deaths related to the big sellers. If millions of patients are taking a drug, sometimes people just die coincidentally while they are on it. Their death could be related to the drug, or an unrelated heart attack. It's only when patterns or frequency appear—as with Prepulsid—that they are required to act."

"What did Health Canada do?" I asked.

"Health Canada sent a letter to Janssen asking for voluntary withdrawal," he explained in a matter-of-fact way. "Janssen said no."

"Why would the people we pay to protect us from dangerous drugs send a letter *asking* a drug company to please stop selling a risky drug?"

"They say they don't have the authority to order a drug off the market."

Michele Brill-Edwards had told me something different: when life is in danger Health Canada doesn't need to negotiate with anyone.[4]

I asked Neil about grapefruit juice.

"It's not just Prepulsid that can cause problems with grapefruit juice. There are a number of drugs that can become toxic with grapefruit juice. We've known that for some time. The antifungal drugs like ketoconazole also cause long QT with Prepulsid. Grapefruit juice inhibits the enzyme P450 CYP3A4 that metabolizes [breaks down] certain drugs.[5] We took grapefruit juice off our hospital menu at Sunnybrook years ago."

That would have gotten the attention of the Oakville doctors.

"What do you remember about the Health Canada meeting you attended in November 1998 where Prepulsid was discussed?"

"The warnings on Prepulsid were unclear. And the label has a lot of small print. There is simply too much information for any busy doctor to read. We call it label clutter. No one reads the labels."

There it was: a problem so common the experts had given it a nickname—label clutter. A drug label could be like a messy room, where you can't find anything. I mentioned the January 2000 Health Canada article. "Do doctors read the Adverse Reaction Newsletter?"

"Well," he shrugged, "it gets mailed to all physicians. But it's not scintillating reading. Most doctors don't read it."

Michele was right. The Prepulsid warning was like a message in a bottle. The number of drug deaths Larry Sasich had described to me had been preying on my mind. Neil was the ideal person to ask about it.

"How many patients actually die from serious adverse reactions in a year?"

"The most comprehensive study on adverse drug reactions was done using U.S. statistics by Lazarou, Pomerantz, and Corey from the University of Toronto published in the *Journal of the American Medical Association* in 1998.[6] They believed it was higher than a hundred thousand a year in hospitals." Just what Larry Sasich had said. Since our population is about one tenth the size, that would mean 10,000 deaths a year in Canadian hospitals.

I spent the next weeks and months researching serious adverse drug reactions. Frankly, I was shocked to discover that after cancer, heart disease, and strokes, adverse drug reactions are the *fourth-leading cause* of death in Canada. Who would have known? And perhaps 39 per cent[7] of all adverse drug reactions in hospitals are *preventable*. Assuming ten thousand hospital deaths a year, if we acted, we could save perhaps four thousand lives a year in hospitals. Some experts believe another ten thousand deaths are caused by prescription drugs *outside* hospitals, including mis-prescribed drugs, errors in administration, and accidental overdoses. Many of these deaths are also preventable.

Two hundred and twenty-nine people died when Swiss Air Flight 111 crashed off the coast of Newfoundland on September 2, 1998. The government of Canada spent over sixty million dollars to find out why. Yet *forty-four times* as many people die from adverse drug reactions in Canadian hospitals every year. That's like a fully loaded Airbus A320 crashing somewhere in Canada every week year-round.[8] Without major improvements in regulation to protect patients it will get worse.

"How often are life-threatening drugs being prescribed for non-life-threatening illnesses?" I asked Neil.

He paused to think. "Off the top of my head, the antihistamines—like Seldane. And Prepulsid."

This was incredibly frustrating for me. Exasperated, I asked, "Prepulsid was killing people under a growing number of conditions. Instead of changing the label five times, and issuing letters that few doctors read, why didn't someone just pull it off the market?" His candid reply has tormented me ever since.

"In the drug industry, killing people is not bad for business. As long as it's not too many."

I HAD BURIED MYSELF KNEE DEEP in Big Pharma's sordid inner workings almost immediately after Vanessa died. By September I was up to my neck. Yet I was still having a problem coming to terms with a shocking fact: the people we trusted with our health and lives apparently had decided it was acceptable for thousands of patients to die taking the medicines administered to help them.

I met with our lawyers on a cool evening—September 5th in Jeremy Taylor's boardroom. We had two weeks to file our lawsuit if we were going to include Health Canada. We still hadn't fully worked out our relationship, but Jeremy and Gary were with us, and that was enough at the time. I told them this drug safety issue was far bigger than Prepulsid. We had to expose the breakdown of the drug surveillance system.

Gary was supportive. "You'll have a chance to advise the inquest jury on how to avoid similar deaths. But we want the inquest to focus on Prepulsid, and the lack of anything like a black box warning for Canadian patients."

Gary was looking at a Canadian Prepulsid "Information for the Patient" pamphlet (October 1999) and comparing it with the U.S. Patient Medication Guide Jeremy picked up in Buffalo. In tiny print with no bold warnings the Canadian one read: "PREPULSID generally has very few side effects." In the eleventh paragraph it warned patients to not exceed the prescribed dose, with no reason given why. It mentioned that Prepulsid should not be used in children, or if "you have a rare ECG abnormality known as QT prolongation (sometimes this runs in families)" or a very slow heart rate. Then it listed the usual drugs and conditions saying only they "should be avoided" and read "You should not take Prepulsid with grapefruit juice." "Not" was underlined.

Gary pointed out the differences: "American patients were told in bold print: serious irregular heartbeats may cause death; stop taking the drug and get medical help if you feel faint; don't take Prepulsid if you have an eating disorder, low electrolytes, persistent vomiting, or your body has lost a lot of water; and serious adverse events, including death, had been reported in children on Prepulsid."

Jeremy said what I was thinking. "It's like they are talking about two different drugs."

Jeremy had researched a 1986 Canadian legal case which had similar facts to ours: Buchan v. Ortho Pharmaceutical (Canada) Ltd. In 1986, after an eleven-year legal battle, an Ontario mother—Pauline Jane Buchan—had been awarded $606,795 in damages upheld by the Ontario Court of Appeals. A non-smoker in excellent health, Pauline had suffered a stroke after taking a birth control drug for six weeks that left her partially paralyzed with brain damage. Jeremy explained that "manufacturers have a duty to provide consumers with an adequate, clear, and understandable warning of dangers inherent in the use of its products. But with prescription drugs, that warning can be through a 'learned intermediary'—a doctor. In Buchan v. Ortho, U.S. doctors were warned in writing about the risk of stroke with Ortho-Novum, and nothing Canadian doctors received even *mentioned* the risk of stroke."

Gary concluded: "Ortho lost because they had no good explanation for the difference in the U.S. and Canadian warnings."

"That sounds very close to our case," I said. "It's even the same company that markets Prepulsid—Johnson & Johnson."

"It's helpful," Gary agreed. "But the devil is in the details. There will be arguments that Vanessa's doctors were given the same information as U.S. doctors about Prepulsid. Our case may depend on how clear and understandable the warnings were."

I knew that any damages for care, guidance, and companionship would be limited, but I was hoping to make our mark for Vanessa in the media with a long public trial and large court award. I asked Gary what out chances were.

"Punitive damages are the only way. But they're very hard

to win. A jury would have to decide the defendants knew, or ought to have known their actions could lead to this."

I interrupted. "I believe I can prove that."

Gary raised his eyebrows and continued ". . . and that the defendants acted maliciously, arbitrarily, or capriciously." There was silence in the room. This was some pretty cryptic legal language. I suspected the courts would have defined these terms. Then it occurred to me I really didn't know Gary that well yet. Maybe he was reconsidering this whole thing.

Finally he broke the silence: "They might view giving Canadians lesser warnings as arbitrary or capricious," he said with a half smile. Gary wasn't quitting. He was relishing the coming fight.

We agreed to meet again in ten days.

EVERYTHING DEPENDED ON A JURY deciding that Prepulsid caused Vanessa's death. Without that, nothing else mattered. The inquest was first, and was the key. I would have one chance at an inquest to make my case: that Vanessa's death was business as usual for a Big Pharma company. Where to start?

I already had over a hundred pages of notes, had dozens of excellent books and articles on the drug industry, and had pieced together a binder quickly filling with studies on the history of Prepulsid. Sometimes late at night, however, I would find myself thinking of Vanessa and I would write down what I wanted to tell the jury as a father. Could I translate the medical-speak and make a jury understand? I was keeping my oath and doing my utmost to be the good guy. But I was fighting a fearsome thought somewhere in the back of my mind, an awareness that sometimes, no matter what, the good guy loses.

I first met Alan Cassels and Colleen Fuller on a sunny morning at the Intercontinental Hotel on Bloor Street in

Toronto. They are co-founders of PharmaWatch in Vancouver, an advocacy group focused on prescription drug safety. Alan was an independent health policy consultant, and Colleen is an advocate who was diabetic and almost died after taking synthetic insulin. Both are passionate about increasing safety for patients and exposing to the public the risks related to prescription drugs.[9] They had followed news of Vanessa's story in the media and asked to meet me when they were in Toronto. We sat and drank coffee at the hotel restaurant while we talked. At this meeting and in later conversations Alan shared his knowledge of the drug industry.

I asked Alan how he got involved in prescription drug safety.

"In 1994 I was doing research on drug pricing for the federal government at the University of British Columbia and found a book at the Ministry of Health library, *The Real Pushers: A Critical Analysis of the Canadian Drug Industry*, by Dr. Joel Lexchin. It was a page turner for me. Joel was way ahead of the curve on Big Pharma tactics. I had no idea this stuff was going on. His examples came from the sixties and seventies, but thirty years later little has changed."

"How powerful are the drug companies?" I asked.

"They're almost omnipotent."

I immediately assumed he was exaggerating. "What do you mean?"

"They use their wealth to influence every agency or organization that influences prescription drugs. That includes governments, professional organizations, associations, coalitions, and patient support groups. They use research dollars and corporate donations to set the agenda at our universities for most health-related research. They control what is studied. It's hard to overstate their influence on our health."

"The official number of deaths related to Prepulsid was

eighty when Vanessa died," I told him. "It's off the open market in Canada and the U.S. Yet they're still selling Prepulsid in many countries."

"Any CEO's first responsibility is to increase shareholder value. That means sales. The problem is the industry is rife with deception. Too often they say one thing, and the truth turns out to be something else. They say they are our doctor's partners in our health care. They'll say this drug is safe, but data later shows that it wasn't really safe. And they *knew* it wasn't safe. Prepulsid is just one of many examples."

"How can they ethically continue to sell risky drugs?"

"The CEO must act to maximize shareholder value by law. Pharmaceutical company profits are head and shoulders above other industries, and have been for years. They'd stop selling risky drugs if it affected their profits. But it doesn't. There is actually no law against it. They follow the law."

I was stunned to hear that there is no law against knowingly selling risky drugs to patients. I had always assumed that there was a statute somewhere that forbade that. But the idea that the law might actually *require* CEOs to keep selling risky blockbusters turned my stomach.

I thought back to Johnson & Johnson's credo. "What about responsibility to patients?"

"Pharmaceutical companies are not health consultants. Their mandate is to sell drugs. They don't make any money unless they do. Legally, responsibility to patients is the doctors' mandate." Jane Cooper's words came back to me: "*The official industry position is that it's up to the doctor and pharmacist to supply the information to patients. It's high-level finger-pointing.*"

"I just don't understand how anyone could do business like that."

"Neither do I. Maybe it would be different if the CEOs had to face the people harmed by their products. But they're so detached—usually in another city or country. In Joel Lexchin's book he refers to drug companies that protected themselves in the sixties against charges by establishing a Vice-President of Going to Jail. It was pre-arranged that one employee would accept responsibility for illegal corporate acts, and be taken care of financially if he ever had to do time. They needn't have bothered. I've never heard of any pharmaceutical company executive in jail. They always end up just paying fines."

"So who is Big Pharma accountable to?"

"Their shareholders. They are truly international companies. The CEO might be in New Jersey or Europe. The drug gets tested in Africa. The pills are made in Puerto Rico, and then sold out of Canadian headquarters in Montreal. There is no loyalty to any country."

"Maybe I'm naive, but I find it hard to believe the Canadian CEOs don't intervene to improve the level of safety on prescription drugs in their own country."

"Canadian CEOs are like franchise managers. They focus on sales, and deal with politicians and regulators. I've never heard of a Canadian subsidiary unilaterally sending out truly effective warnings or voluntarily pulling a drug off the market before a regulator really puts the pressure on."

That would be *after* too many patients died, from what I'd been told. My thoughts went back to the inquest and our lawsuit. Dr. Joel Lexchin might make a good witness for us.

"Did the industry take Joel Lexchin to court to try and silence him?"

"They couldn't, because his work is all evidence-based. He's got data to back up everything he writes. Talk to Joel. In critical analysis of the pharmaceutical industry, he's a giant."

Alan described the Big Pharma companies as almost omnipotent. Late that night I found a similar statement in a book that had held me entranced—*Bitter Pills*, by Stephen Fried.

Fried's wife, Diane Ayers, had suffered a serious adverse reaction in 1997 after taking another Johnson & Johnson drug, antibiotic Floxin. An industry insider had described Big Pharma power to Fried: "the big companies are not American, or German or Canadian—they are countries unto themselves."[10]

Transfer pricing was described to Fried as the cornerstone of pharmaceutical price gouging.[11] Trade agreements allowed the Big Pharma companies to manufacture the drug chemicals in one country, and then buy them from themselves at a huge markup to be bottled in another country. Profits were moved to a low tax jurisdiction. It's a legal form of tax avoidance. But it also meant that Big Pharma CEOs could shut down facilities in any country—or threaten to—if local regulators or politicians became too annoying.

I recalled a conversation I'd had with a Big Pharma rep when I was MPP. He'd been telling me how head office in Europe was considering building a new plant just a few miles away in Mississauga, providing three hundred new jobs; then immediately proceeded to outline why their newest drug should be placed on the Ontario formulary. The plant and the jobs created was the carrot. Or its cancellation could be a stick.

Fried also recounted the tale of Retin-A, another Johnson & Johnson drug out of their Ortho division. In 1996 Ortho had paid $7.5 million to the FDA in a plea bargain arrangement to settle ten criminal counts of obstruction of justice and cover FDA costs. This followed an eight-year FDA investigation of the promotional practices at Johnson & Johnson and Ortho. Ortho employees had secretly shredded documents related to off-label promotion of Retin-A, and Johnson & Johnson ended up pleading guilty to obstructing justice for destroying them, avoiding a potential penalty of double the revenues earned from illegal acts—a possible $1 billion.

The story troubled me deeply because Prepulsid had been

prescribed widely off-label—for infants and for teens with bloating. Where did Dr. Kayner hear that this was a good idea? And it painted a disturbing picture for me: people standing around an office shredder feeding in documents a government agency had ordered their employer to produce.

Were the Big Pharma companies really like countries unto themselves?

I had to find out. And I never went wrong following the money. From 1991 the pharmaceutical industry made more money than software, hardware, energy, mining—everything, with profits averaging about 30 per cent of revenues.[12] The top Big Pharma companies had more annual sales revenue than the gross national product of over a hundred countries in the world.

How did they get so wealthy?

The *Wall Street Journal* reported in July 2001 that most Big Pharma companies spent on average twice as much on marketing and administration than on research and development, a fact that staggered me. Some even had profits bigger than their R&D budget. Based on spending, marketing was their business, and R&D was secondary.

And the marketing worked. By 2000 Canadians were spending more on drugs than we did on doctors—15.5 per cent of our total health expense. Drug expenses were 17 per cent in 2007.

The largest international pharmaceutical companies have their head offices outside Canada, mostly in the U.S. So top executives in other countries make decisions critical to Canadian health and safety. But what undermines our safety with drugs more than anything else is that they must consider the interests of their international shareholders first. That is why it is totally inappropriate for Health Canada to "partner" with the drug companies. When sales and safety conflict, sales win, and people get hurt.

Big Pharma CEOs can move their head offices or plants almost anywhere in the world; pack up their jobs and leave. Their investments are always welcome elsewhere. And they make sure our elected officials never forget that.[13] With that kind of leverage, it's no wonder that drugs increase every year not just in number, but in price.

As the ultimate authority for issuing warnings, post market studies and keeping risky drugs on the market, foreign executives literally have power over life and death for Canadians. This is more power than any other individual, other than perhaps a prime minister or president. But political leaders are accountable to the other branches of government, the voters, and their parties. To whom are Big Pharma CEOs accountable?

We recently saw former executives from Enron, Adelphia Communications, and Worldcom go to prison for financial crimes. Yet apparently no one at Merck, makers of Vioxx—a drug ultimately responsible for 120,000 heart attacks and strokes and as many as 56,000 deaths—faced any sanctions. Raymond Gilmartin, the former president and CEO, still held a position of honour there two years later.[14] The man who was in charge at Johnson & Johnson during the nineties when the Prepulsid label was changed five times and off-label sales kept rising—Ralph S. Larson—remained as chairman until 2002. In short, when people die after taking risky drugs, no one at Big Pharma goes to jail. Numerous deaths and injuries don't appear to even hurt their careers.

Drugs that are dangerous under numerous conditions are widely prescribed and sold. The word "dangerous," like "safe," is a matter of degree. There is no law requiring warnings to be proven effective. Warnings are a matter of negotiation. And I've never discovered any significant sanction against a Big Pharma company for breaking promises made to governments to conduct safety studies. Someday, and I hope it's not a long way off, we'll look back at this time for what it is—the Wild West of human health, and wonder how we let it go on.

Perhaps the most important thing I learned during those late nights was that drugs and health are not one in the same. You don't always need drugs. Many of the ailments we suffer from are diseases caused by drugs, and we don't even know it. Some "cures" can kill. So taking the right drug at the right time, or not taking a drug, is an incredibly important decision. It's that simple.

Chapter 10

This Business of Disease

"When money speaks, the truth keeps silent."
—Russian proverb

THE MORE I READ, the more I discovered that people were taking an awful lot of drugs they didn't need, and often couldn't afford. Why so many?

Anna Kovacs had read about the coming inquest and had called me to extend her condolences. She was an industry insider I had met back in 1995. I met Anna for lunch in Toronto. It turns out she decided to leave the drug manufacturer she had worked for and was now working as a corporate consultant. I asked her about the drug industry. Anna was brutally frank.

"Vanessa's death was a result of how the drug industry operates. People are given too many drugs. They see that as normal. We want a pill for every ill because of TV advertising, and because of what physicians are prescribing. We are over-medicated. It's ludicrous, and it can be dangerous."

"Why do doctors write so many prescriptions?"

"They want to help patients—to treat them. But they throw

drugs at most problems. They hand patients a free sample, and patients are obedient. They try it and all come back and say it worked."

"You mean sometimes drugs *don't* work?"

"Some drugs don't work on some patients. Most conditions go away on their own anyway. The patients think it was the drug that helped them. They believe it, so the doctors believe it. Who's to tell them otherwise?"

I remembered Vanessa saying that she thought Prepulsid helped her. But had it really? If it hadn't helped, she had died for no reason.

"Vanessa was prescribed Prepulsid off-label."

"Off-label is the way of the world. With some drugs, off-label use is more common than approved use. For example, Imitrex [to treat migraine]. It's not proven safe to use more than four times in thirty days—four headaches—one pill each time. Yet some doctors write out prescriptions for thirty pills at a time. Migraine is so painful, patients often take more."

I remembered what Michele Brill-Edwards had said about Imitrex, that it had a narrow therapeutic index. Not a drug you should double dose.

"Don't the doctors know better?"

Anna leaned forward for emphasis: "The doctors don't get the proper information to evaluate risk. Yet they are the real decision-makers—Big Pharma's real customer. All the company's marketing efforts are focused on getting the doctors to write their name on a prescription pad. They do it with free samples, gifts, consulting fees, whatever it takes. There are doctors in Toronto eating lobster every night on the drug companies' dime."

"What does the government do about all this?"

"Governments *pay*. The Ontario Drug Benefit Plan is the largest single drug buyer in North America. And they can be a thorn in Big Pharma's side. They decide which drugs get on the

Ontario formularies. To get a drug approved for sale, the pharmaceutical companies only have to show Health Canada it works better than a placebo. But to get the provinces to *pay* for it, they have to show it works better than a drug already on the formulary. Big difference."

"Can you give me an example?"

"Sure, omeprazole," she said. "It's the generic name for AstraZeneca's blockbuster for heartburn, Losec—the 'purple pill.'[1] Ontario paid over $70 million last year for Losec. Its patents will expire next year and generics will be available for a lot less. But AstraZeneca got a patent approved for esomeprazole (Nexium), a me-too derivative, to keep their customers paying brand prices for another purple pill. They're pushing to get it on the formulary. Ontario said no, repeatedly."

This strategy was similar to what Johnson & Johnson had done with Prepulsid after Motilium.

"How high are the markups on drugs?"

Anna raised her eyebrows and sighed. "High! I've seen markups anywhere from 30 per cent to 96 per cent in Canada. The Patented Medicine Prices Review Board sets the prices— another source of frustration to the companies—because it keeps prices in Canada much lower than U.S. prices. Canadians end up paying about median prices worldwide."

"What about transfer pricing—buying the drugs from themselves off-shore to reduce taxes?"

"You're thinking of the manufacturer's cost of active ingredients. It's almost impossible to find out what they pay. It's become the subject of urban myth. But the cost of the ingredients has absolutely no relationship to the price the patient pays at the pharmacy. The drug companies set prices as high as they can get away with. With Imitrex they asked themselves: how much will people pay to get rid of a fierce headache? And that became the price."

"Generic drug prices are far lower, right?"

"They usually cost about half, sometimes more, but their markups are still high enough for them to pay half or more of the purchase price *back* to pharmacists. Some people call it rebates. Most people would call it kickbacks."

This bothered me. I thought back to my first job at age seventeen in a Bata shoe store. We were paid a $2 bonus for selling "spiffs"—styles that were poor sellers. Other industries have internal incentives for salespeople, like the auto industry. But a pharmacist is a trusted healthcare professional, not a shoe salesman.

I asked Anna about "breakthrough drugs."

She chuckled. "Over 90 per cent of new drugs are me-too drugs—like the fifth cholesterol-lowering drug—or 'evergreen' drugs—like faster acting versions of a pill, or pills you take once a day instead of three times. Look at Losec. The government of Canada actually gave AstraZeneca a new patent for taking the active ingredient in the pill and putting it in a *capsule*."

"But their websites and magazine ads show people in lab coats gazing into test tubes. They talk about cures." Anna's voice dripped with disdain. "They aren't looking for cures. If they stumble across one, they'll market it."

IF THE MARKUPS ON PRESCRIPTION DRUGS ranged from 30 per cent to 96 per cent, that would explain why Big Pharma companies had profits multiple those of other industries. But if they were spending two to three times as much on marketing and administration as R&D, where did that money go?

One place I discovered was executive compensation. I was staggered to learn that in 2000 the top five remuneration packages for drug company executives ranged from $19 million to $40 million, with unexercised stock options from $81 million to $227 million,[2]—between hundreds and thousands of times the average industrial wage. By 2007 five of the top Big Pharma CEOs earned from $19 to $33 million.[3]

Each drug patent is a government-granted monopoly, for which the drug companies can charge whatever they want. But drugs are not photocopiers or cameras. Many of them are critical for human health and well-being. And I'd read reports, including one from Congresswoman Carolyn Maloney of New York, that some U.S. patients were forced to cut their pills in half to be able to afford their drugs.[4]

Governments grant drug patents to encourage research for breakthroughs. But governments in Canada are the ones paying the most for these drugs, like Ontario's 2000 Losec bill at $70 million. In December 2006 Pfizer president, Canadian-born Hank McKinnell, was shown the door and given a financial package worth $190 million.[5]

I imagine that some of the folks who struggle to pay Pfizer's prices would find it hard to even imagine that much money. Why give drug companies monopolies for "evergreening"—minor variations on existing drugs—when all that does is keep the prices of the active ingredients so high that Big Pharma CEOs can afford luxury yachts?

SO WHAT HAVE BIG PHARMA CEOS and a "pill for every ill" done for our health? How healthy are we? Well, Canadians take an average of fourteen prescriptions a year. Yet for overall health the World Health Organization places Canada in thirtieth place, and the U.S.—whose citizens take slightly more prescription drugs—at thirty-seventh.

And billions of dollars are wasted. The Canadian Pharmacist's Association says that the cost of under use, misuse, and overuse of prescription drugs could range *between $2 billion* *and $9 billion a year.*[6] How much healthier would Canadians be if we invested that money in preventative health care, things like regular checkups, physical activity, stress management, diet education, tobacco intervention, and tests like pap smears and colonoscopies?

By 2001, in addition to a great deal of human misery, drug errors cost our healthcare system a staggering $10.9 billion a year.[7] Every time a drug injures a patient we all pay. Prescription drugs are related to *one out of four hospital admissions* for internal medicine patients—for things like things like heart, respiratory, gastrointestinal, and kidney problems.[8] Up to 60 per cent of those admissions may be preventable.

I wondered if Anna Kovacs had been totally fair about Big Pharma stumbling across cures. Late one night while Googling "cures" I came across this suggestion on a medical chat forum: "Try this party game some time. Ask if anyone can name a drug, outside of antibiotics, that cures a disease." I went blank. I couldn't think of one. But I was determined to find out if there were any.

Late September 2000

Sometimes between appointments I would visit Vanessa's grave at Mount Pleasant Cemetery, a beautiful and peaceful sanctuary in Toronto. Surrounded by a hundred different kinds of trees and flora, it's a sacred place to many of its visitors. Occasionally I'd find faded flowers that Vanessa's friends had left at her grave with signed notes or letters. I was awed at how Vanessa's life and soul had touched so many friends, and how loyal those friends were to her now. In my mind I often pictured how she and her friends had greeted each other—always with a hug. Those teenagers were truly beautiful. They really gave me hope for the future.

One sunny September afternoon I turned off Mount Pleas-ant Avenue to enter the cemetery and saw a row of unmarked white transport trailers parked along the curb. Inside, blocking the road, were two young people wearing baseball caps and blue jeans, drinking coffee out of cardboard cups and chatting. I asked them what was up.

"We're filming a movie."

"Where?"

"Just over there, at the crematorium."

This seemed strangely inappropriate. I was immediately suspicious. "What kind of movie?" I asked.

"A rock musical."

A rock musical. Maybe it was the look in their eyes. But I doubted it. I wasn't against filming at the cemetery. The Massey family had approved filming part of the classic series *Anne of Green Gables* at the Massey Mausoleum a few years before. Great. But I was wary; these people might be shooting some schlocky horror movie. As I drove over to the Toronto Trust Cemeteries office on the grounds, I saw a two-sided sign standing on the sidewalk: "Filming Isabella Rocks."

The manager was in.

"Mr. Young," the well-dressed manager assured me, "I read every script before giving anyone permission to film on the grounds." So they'd done this before.

"B movie scripts can change at any time." I said. "How much is the cemetery getting paid for this?" He could have told me to get stuffed.

"There are fees for filming in the cemetery," he replied diplomatically.

I admit I was on a slow boil. Cemeteries are licenced by the province of Ontario to be operated in trust for burials, a place for family members to commune with the spirits of their loved ones in a dignified atmosphere. That licence did not include turning a cemetery into a profit centre. What *else* might they be doing for extra cash? I wondered.

I suppose I was being overly protective. But looking back, I think it was because the pursuit of money over what is sacred— human life—was the reason I was at the cemetery in the first place. And I'd lost my trust in institutions. If I couldn't protect Vanessa in life, at least I'd protect her resting place.

It later turned out my instincts were right. The film was released for TV in 2001 under the name *Murder Among Friends*.

Alan Cassels had described Dr. Joel Lexchin as a giant in critical analysis of the pharmaceutical industry. What does a giant look like? Joel is 5'7" and, despite a walking disability as a result of contracting polio as a child, dons his windbreaker and knapsack year round and rides his bicycle to work at the Emergency at Toronto's University Health Network. He also conducts research as Associate Chair of the York University School of Health Policy and Management in matters such as drug safety, approvals, promotion, prices, and pharmacare.[9] His research has been published in medical journals around the world.

We communicated mostly by telephone and email, and his replies were always thoughtful and detailed. I asked Joel about cures.

"Does Big Pharma cure diseases?"

"It depends on your definition of a cure. Vaccines prevent disease and are highly valuable when used properly. There used to be thousands of cases of polio in Canada in the 1950s. I was one of them. Now we don't have any. Smallpox is now eliminated worldwide. Other drugs make treatments possible. If you break your hip and need surgery, it wouldn't be possible without anesthetics."

"But when someone says cure, I always envision a disease being reversed, gone."

"Infectious diseases like strep and pneumonia have been cured by antibiotics, cured in the sense that the individual who has the infection gets better. However, the disease itself has not been eliminated: people continue to get pneumonia and strep throat."

That immediately brought back a memory—one night when Vanessa was two years old and running a fever due to an ear infection, Dr. Kayner had actually come to our house to diagnose her and prescribe an antibiotic. Within hours her fever was down, like a miracle. Antibiotics helped Madeline and Hart as well. But antibiotics were developed in the early 1940s, sixty years before.

"I was thinking of more recent innovations," I said.

"About 80 per cent of children with acute lymphoblastic leukemia are cured. Other non-solid forms of cancer are very treatable and lives are extended. With cancer, one definition of cure is when you are treated for cancer and later die from something else with no evidence of cancer. A more meaningful word might be breakthroughs. These cancer drugs would be considered medical breakthroughs."

In 2000 eighty-one new human drugs had been introduced for sale in Canada. In June of 2001 the people who help determine what prescription drugs will sell for in Canada—the Patented Medicines Price Review Board—published their 2000 Annual Report, placing those drugs in three categories: comparable form of an existing medicine; one with moderate, little or no improvement; and substantial improvement or "breakthrough." *Only three of eighty-one new drugs were identified as breakthroughs.* And none of the three breakthroughs claimed to be a cure.

From 1996–2000 only 5 per cent of drugs introduced in Canada were breakthroughs or substantial improvements.[10]

If we accept the broadest possible definition of "cure,"

which includes preventing disease, or extending life, cures are still less than 5 per cent of what Big Pharma comes up with. The drug companies do look for cures, but if your definition of cure means eliminating a disease state in a patient like antibiotics do, they haven't discovered any in decades.

Which left me with a question: If less than 5 per cent of your new products are cures and breakthroughs, and over 95 per cent of them treat disease by comparable or moderate improvement, what business are you really in—the cures business or the disease business?

As I told various friends about the 110,000 deaths in U.S. and Canadian hospitals from adverse drug reactions, and additional deaths outside hospitals, I began to realize they were thinking one of two things: "this poor guy has lost it," or "if this true, why am I hearing it for the first time"? I asked Joel about those numbers.

"The Lazarou study concluded that they are one hundred thousand in-hospital deaths a year due to adverse reactions when prescription drugs are taken as prescribed. Nobody knows how many additional deaths there are in the community from adverse reactions, including things like prescribing errors, dispensing errors, and unidentified overdoses. Some researchers assume an additional one hundred thousand deaths a year—one death for every 1500 people a year in the U.S."

That would mean the total number of U.S. deaths due to adverse drug reactions could be 200,000 a year, and adverse drug reactions as high as 2 million.

"But you should know not all adverse drug reactions are preventable," Joel continued. "Some drug-related deaths are from treatments where the patient would have died without treatment. And some could not be predicted. There are different estimates about the percentage of adverse drug reactions that are preventable, ranging from about 35 to about 60 per cent."

That could mean seventy thousand to a hundred and twenty thousand deaths that may be preventable in the U.S. I asked Joel about Canada.

"We often use a 10 per cent figure based on our population. So it could be as high as twenty thousand ADR deaths in Canada a year. But the short answer is, no one knows."

That would be more deaths than all vehicular accidents, homicides, accidental falls, and war put together.

I reminded Joel about the five label changes for Prepulsid. His answer was like a kick in the gut. "Warnings make little difference in the prescribing habits of doctors," he said matter-of-factly.

"What do you mean?" I managed to say.

"In the mid nineteen-eighties in the U.S., despite label changes and warnings that encainide [Enkaid] and flecainide [Tambocor] were causing heart arrhythmias and were related to 50,000 deaths, yet 80 per cent of specialists who responded to a survey continued prescribing them to the same patients. In 1983, after the painkiller zompirac [Zomax] was related to numerous deaths due to anaphylaxis, label changes and warnings letters to doctors had no impact on its use. It was withdrawn. Canadian data also tells us warnings don't affect prescribing."

JOHNSON & JOHNSON'S POSITION had always been that they had changed the label on Prepulsid five times since 1995 to reduce inappropriate prescribing. During that time Prepulsid sales continued to climb. They must have watched what happened with Tambocor and Enkaid—one of the worst drug disasters in history. Not only that, Zomax had been a Johnson & Johnson drug. They'd been through this before—a new drug, deadly adverse reactions, label changes, more deadly adverse reactions, and finally drug withdrawal. After the Buchan v. Ortho lawsuit and Zomax, Johnson & Johnson officials would be well aware of any ongoing study on adverse drug reactions caused by one of their blockbusters.

If anyone knew that label changes didn't much affect pre-ocribing ratco, it would be the people at Johnson & Johnson.

One evening I spent hours on the Internet Googling "cisapride" and "warnings" and found a U.S. study that been done on Prepulsid from June 1998 to June 1999, *after* the fourth label change and the black box warning had been added. In the year before, 26 to 58 per cent of Prepulsid users at three health centres were already at risk for heart arrhythmias or were taking drugs that were contraindicated with Prepulsid. In the year *after* the warnings that number only fell by only 2 per cent.[11] That study confirmed that the Prepulsid warnings to doctors were virtually useless, and by 1999, *24 to 56 per cent of Prepulsid users were taking the drug when it wasn't safe.*

The lead researcher, Dr. Walter Smalley of Vanderbilt University had called it a breakdown of the healthcare system.

A lot of Prepulsid sales were off-label. "How much prescribing of other drugs is off-label?" I asked Joel.

"It is difficult to say. Not all off-label prescribing is bad. If the company chooses *not* to add indications to a drug's label then even well-accepted uses will continue to be off-label. Back in 1992 Health Canada surveyed two hundred doctors on a range of issues, including how often they prescribe off-label. The results were: frequently, 6 per cent; sometimes, 26 per cent; not too often, 41 per cent; and never, 25 per cent."

Seventy three per cent of doctors prescribed off-label—the riskiest kind of prescribing—even back in 1992 before the big blockbuster boom of the nineties.

But as Joel said, a company could choose to not add "indications" to a drug label. Of course! Why bother going through all the delays and hassle of getting the FDA and Health Canada to approve a new "indication" as safe, when you could easily use the Wild West approach—persuade almost three out of four doctors in their offices to write millions of off-label prescriptions?

Then Joel summarized the safest way to introduce a new drug, one of the most important statements I'd heard since Vanessa died: "Unless a drug is a really major advance, it should be used very cautiously for the first few years. Give it to people who reflect the group it was tested on. If drugs are introduced gradually then hopefully serious side effects will be picked up early and we can avoid exposing large numbers of people to them. Hopefully is the operative word here because we need a good post-marketing surveillance system, which we don't have."

Alex Demerse had told me doctors don't report adverse drug reactions because they don't want to be sued, no doubt a key reason. A report might be used in court as evidence of malpractice. From what I'd heard, when patients experience adverse reactions many doctors will just switch them to a different drug. Assuming the patient is still alive. Doctors say ADRs are hard to identify. But there are other reasons doctors don't want to report them. And as time went on I began to discover that doctors would fight the idea of mandatory ADR reporting right to the end.

"Serious ADRs are underreported, but it will take a sea change to get doctors to *routinely* report ADRs," Joel advised me. "We don't need to know that someone given ampicillin has developed a rash that went away after the drug was stopped. But any reaction that is unexpected [not previously known] should be reported. And every rare but serious reaction should be reported. We need to know the frequency of serious reactions. Since they occur much less frequently, there is more hope of getting doctors to report these."

I was doubtful. "Most doctors I've met have never reported an ADR, even a serious one."

"Rare serious reactions may be commonly known, but doctors and pharmacists feel that since the reaction is known, there is no reason for further reports. This type of reasoning is a mistake, since the reason that a reaction may be 'rare' is that it is infrequently reported."

Mistake? Joel had a remarkable tendency to make very important statements in a matter-of-fact way. This was definitely where the rubber hit the road for me: doctors who know a life-threatening reaction might happen, don't realize that how *often* it happens to patients could be lifesaving information for others? If every adverse reaction to Prepulsid had been reported, and Health Canada didn't withhold the information like they did with Sana's report, I believed Prepulsid would have been off the market long before it was prescribed to Vanessa.

Maybe the choice for doctors between reporting that their medical intervention harmed a patient, and pretending nothing happened, was too easy to make. If they didn't report them, who would ever know?

I asked one of my new contacts, Carol Kushner, co-author (with Michael Rachlis) of two books on our medical system—*Strong Medicine* and *Second Opinion*—her view of the claim that ADRs aren't reported because they're hard to identify.

"I don't buy that. Let's err on the side of caution. If it's serious, make the report: 'This drug may have been contributory.' The importance will emerge if it turns out the ADR is not isolated. Once a deadly side effect is recognized you can get a drug off the market."

"I've heard that some doctors didn't report ADRs because they feel nothing meaningful is done with them," I told Carol.

She was sympathetic. "Mandatory reporting with no follow-up is worse than useless. It creates cynicism. I support it as long as Health Canada is doing something with them, and as long as patient reports continued to be analyzed and valued. They are rich with detail."

"Some doctors say they don't have time to report."

"I've heard that. One doctor told me he saw ten suspected ADRs a day and if he had to report them it would take him two and a half hours. But there are ways around that."

Carol was right, in my view. Almost every doctor has Internet access or a fax machine. How long would it take to fill out a one page form entitled *Suspected Adverse Drug Reaction* and send it along to a drug SWAT team at Health Canada? The combined observations of the entire medical profession would help spot new risks, or deadly reactions like those from thalidomide or Prepulsid, in months, instead of years.

Carol summed up the doctors' dilemma, lowering her voice almost to a whisper, "There's another reason that no one talks about. I think it must be quite devastating to give a drug to a patient to help them, and find out it harmed them."

AS I READ MORE I LEARNED that new drugs are definitely not introduced slowly. Blockbuster sales are driven by billions of dollars' worth of direct-to-consumer advertising, and sophisticated marketing techniques designed to get as many patients as possible to take the drug now. And to make the decision to do so while looking at the ad—long before they even see their doctor.

I spent a lot of time on the investor websites, like www.forbes.com, and read investor blogs. Many investors bet on drugs in the Big Pharma development pipeline becoming blockbusters like gamblers bet on horses. This makes drugs a commodity like pork bellies, and helps ensure that developing drugs for chronic conditions, not cures, is Big Pharma's priority. The longer the patient's condition lasts, the longer they'll need the drug, and the greater the return on investment.

Reading investor chat pages made me realize that chronic diseases make people an awful lot of money. Cures are the last thing markets want. Return on investment, not what's good for patients, even drives what drugs are developed in the pipeline. Drugs that treat acute diseases—those that last a short time—rarely develop into blockbusters. In fact many acute diseases are no longer "cost-effective." One round of a good antibiotic and your infection can be gone. Some companies are getting right out of making potentially lifesaving antibiotic drugs, and the number of them available is dropping.

The stakes are very high. For example, if an easy, cheap, and safe way was discovered to lower high cholesterol today, Pfizer would have $14 billion a year in Lipitor sales at risk. If Lipitor was pulled off the market Pfizer could end up in the red in short order.[12] In December 2006 Pfizer's most promising pipeline drug—torcetrapib—was discovered in clinical trials to cause heart problems and deaths, and its market development was cancelled. Pfizer's share price fell by more than 11 per cent, reducing its total market value by US $21 billion. One announcement—$21 billion.

For Big Pharma to prioritize a drug it must be cost-effective. That means there must be a very large disease population who lives in countries where people can pay for the drugs. That's why only 10 per cent of global research (private and public combined) is devoted to diseases that account for 90 per cent of the world's disease burden.[13] Malaria, measles, and diarrhea are diseases that are not cost-effective in Africa today, which means if people contract them there they will probably die. Chronic diseases or conditions that attract Big Pharma drug development are cancer, hypertension (high blood pressure), psychiatric disorders (depression is the biggest), rheumatoid arthritis (arthritis of the joints), and thrombosis (blood clots).[14]

Drugs that treat patients' conditions in developed nations—

like erectile dysfunction and the granddaddy blockbuster condition of them all, higher than average cholesterol[15]—draw big blockbuster action. The U.S. market for drugs that lower cholesterol (statins) was $27 billion in 2006. "Orphan" diseases—the least cost-effective—are rare diseases for which potential cures are available, but have no profit potential. They simply are not developed unless governments get involved.[16]

The original purpose of medicines, to heal the sick, has been twisted. They've become commercial commodities that must be widely marketed and sold at huge markups to support large bureaucracies, compensate some of the highest-paid executives in the world, and to pay dividends to shareholders. Things that get in the way of the marketing machines—like patient safety—are expendable. Some of the marketing tactics I uncovered were distasteful. Others were downright deceptive. Here are few examples:

Big Pharma marketers will argue on end that their copycat drug is different and better than the original. What they don't talk about is that similar drugs can cause similar side effects. Cialis is marketed to be longer-acting than Viagra. But Cialis and Viagra (and all drugs in their class) present serious risks to anyone taking nitrates or with low blood pressure. Hundreds of men have died after taking Viagra. And both drugs have warnings about sudden hearing loss and even permanent blindness.

Celebrex (celecoxib) is similar to Vioxx (both are COX-2 inhibitors) and may also carry the risk of heart attack and strokes.[17] Another COX-2 inhibitor—Bextra (valdecoxib)—has already been pulled off the market for damaging patient's livers.

Cholesterol drug Baycol was pulled off the market for causing a dangerous muscle wasting condition called rhabdomyolysis. That same awful side effect can be caused by Lipitor, Zocor, Crestor and other statin drugs. But it's not just the similar adverse reactions patients have to watch out for, it's potential new ones—because the copycat molecule is just a little different then the original.

Big Pharma companies actually market their failures. For example, Viagra was originally tested as a heart drug, until someone later noticed the male patients on it developed erections.

Sometimes the drug companies also go back to old molecules (drugs) they own—even if they were taken off the market for harming or killing patients—and repackage them. In other words, they market their mistakes. In 1998 the FDA re-approved thalidomide—responsible for one of the worst drug disasters in history—this time to treat leprosy and multiple myeloma in a restricted access program, and it is being used to treat cancer. The original name thalidomide would strike fear in many patients, so they simply created two new names—Revlimid for cancer or Thalomid for leprosy. Neat trick.

They also market drugs' side effects. Remember the drug Motilium (domperidone) used for stomach problems? For safety reasons it was never approved in the U.S., and Johnson & Johnson took it off the market in Canada in 2002, presumably for causing heart arrhythmias in IV form. One of its side effects is lactation. Even men's breasts can start leaking milk while they are taking Motilium. (That's embarrassing.) So now it's sold to help new mothers lactate. But who is telling new mothers domperidone can cause heart arrhythmias?[18]

Sometimes I began to think Big Pharma would consider selling any drug to anybody. Pfizer has spent a lot of money testing Viagra to improve sexual function for women. Last time I looked, women didn't have … well, you know. Needless to say the tests did not go well, and were abandoned.[19]

Big Pharma sometimes play like the camel from the old Bedouin tale getting inside his master's tent.[20] They'll ask for approval for a new drug to treat a very serious illness where a higher level of risk is acceptable, and get it. Then *later* they request an approval for a less severe condition. And they often get it despite the different risk/benefit ratio. Methotrexate was originally approved to fight cancer, but later sold to treat arthritis. Biphosphonates were approved to control pain from bone metastases and later sold for osteoporosis. It's about lowering the safety bar.

In my research I never uncovered any intent to harm patients at Big Pharma companies. Yet while sales soared, millions had been harmed, and the drug industry seemed callously indifferent. I began to realize that indifference could only prevail if something was missing. One late night as I leaned back in my chair in front of my computer screen I realized what it was: compassion for patients. It was mercy. We are naive to expect mercy to overrule the fantastic financial rewards Big Pharma executives get for successfully marketing blockbusters. It would take a very special kind of CEO to make the decision to pull a blockbuster off the market before he absolutely had to, because out of a million customers, some old people or a handful of children will likely die after taking it. Especially when he faces no personal penalty or sanction for doing so. These guys are not nuns. They don't get paid for mercy. What I'd learned all those late nights at my computer is that Shakespeare was wrong. The quality of mercy *is* strained. It is strained through money.

Chapter 11

Deny. Delay. Divide. Discredit.

"If we don't stand up for children, then we don't stand for much."
—Marian Wright Edelman

ON SEPTEMBER 15, 2000, I met with Gary Will and Jeremy Taylor in Jeremy's boardroom. We were out of time. We had to file our lawsuit within four days, and this was decision day.

Halton Regional Police had completed their investigation. The care Vanessa received after she collapsed was not at issue. The paramedics and doctors at both hospitals had done what was best under the circumstances. The main issue at the inquest and future trial would be: Did Prepulsid cause Vanessa's death?

The media would lose interest, and our civil case would be in serious jeopardy if the inquest jury didn't find Vanessa's death was accidental, and that Prepulsid was the cause.

Alex Demerse and Jane Cooper had told me Vanessa's life was a cost of doing business. Others, like pharmacist Sana

Sukkari led me to believe it would difficult—but not impossible to prove that Prepulsid caused Vanessa's death. "Cause and effect" was the incredibly high scientific standard of proof we faced.

Which would it be—difficult, or impossible? The difference would be between some kind of justice for Vanessa, or a whitewash of her death.

With regards to our civil case, Michele Brill-Edwards had given me a dire warning at Joso's restaurant about Big Pharma: "If they are sued by victims of a deadly drug, first they deny. They never admit anything. Then they exhaust victims with delays—legal motions that take years to iron out, knowing the plaintiffs are emotionally exhausted and need closure. Then, they go quietly to injured victims or the families of deceased victims, and offer deals—cash settlements. When a drug crashes there are usually many of them. But they insist the victims sign a gag order that they will never talk about the case again to anyone. So they divide the plaintiffs up—one by one. If any of the victims refuse to settle, they try to discredit them in court. Deny. Delay. Divide. Discredit. That's what you're facing."

Signing such a "gag order" would be unthinkable for me. I'd been conducting the media interviews to warn others of the risks and make sure the case wasn't forgotten—trying to get something positive out of Vanessa's loss. To stop this work in exchange for money would be betrayal of my oath.

Gary said that punitive damages were our only chance of even getting the attention of the industry. So I was severely deflated to discover that unlike Americans, in class actions Canadians have no right to a jury trial. "While any party to an action has a right to request that the issues be decided by a jury," he told me, "the judge will have overriding discretion to disallow a jury, where the issues in dispute are thought to be too complex. In Canada there has yet to be a class action case which has been decided by a jury."

The lawyers for the other side could argue that our case was too complicated for a jury of our peers to understand. Everything we worked on for years might end up relying on one person, a judge.

With all due respect, judges are human and can make mistakes. And they have biases. What if we got a judge whose father had been a wonderful, dedicated doctor—unfairly sued for malpractice—or his mother a dedicated researcher who had helped find a true breakthrough drug? The doctors and Johnson & Johnson might get a more sympathetic hearing.

Juries make mistakes too, as in Donald Marshall's case, a man who spent eleven years in prison for a murder he didn't commit. But at least with a jury I'd potentially have mothers and fathers hearing what I had learned. I felt I could connect with a jury.

What Gary told me next was even more daunting: any plaintiff that fails to prove their case in court could be ordered to pay the legal costs of the defendants. And the threat of ruinous legal consequences went even further. A plaintiff would have to pay those costs, even if they won the trial and proved the defendant had distributed a dangerous drug which had caused injury. That could happen if the amount awarded by the judge or jury was less than the defendant had offered to pay prior to the trial. So victims could lose a family member to a prescription drug, and then be ordered to pay hundreds of thousands of dollars to the drug company and doctors in costs. We didn't have that kind of money, so if we lost we could be paying the defendants the rest of our lives. And making any deal with those responsible for Vanessa's death was the last thing I wanted to do. I had seen and heard too much. As a former elected official, I had already started a list of regulatory changes that I knew would save lives in Canada. I knew in my heart that Vanessa would be pleased that good might come from her loss. A gag order was out of the question.

Gary raised some possible strategies. "Since Vanessa was taking no other drugs at the time of her death, the lawyers for Johnson & Johnson might pull out all the stops to convince the jury that Vanessa had a lifelong heart problem—congenital long QT. This alleged heart problem would theoretically be what made Vanessa susceptible to heart arrhythmia."

Blame the patient. It didn't matter that there was absolutely no evidence that this was true. All they'd have to do is convince the jury that a heart arrhythmia due to congenital long QT could happen to anyone at any time. This appalled me.

Gary continued "The lawyers for the doctors—the CMPA—might try to convince the jury that Vanessa wasn't throwing up, or had lied about it. If she wasn't throwing up, they could argue Prepulsid made no difference."

This would be even more bizarre. There was no question throwing up was Vanessa's problem. She'd been quite open about it. It was the only reason she'd seen the doctors.

There was one other vital issue I had to face the lawyers with. Contingency fees were normal for class actions. In a class action, Gary and Jeremy had a decent chance of having their fees paid in full, if they won the case. But I wasn't sure at the time whether I could fully commit to a class action.

A class action would be based on what everyone in "the class" had in common: Prepulsid. Since all the victims had different doctors, the doctors could all be off the hook. Doctors were part of the problem. They didn't read drug labels or warning letters from the drug companies. They got their drug information from detail reps. Many doctors were more engaged in the gifts, dinners, and free trips from Big Pharma than studying patient safety.[1] For me, the medical profession had lost its way. I wanted to expose their lack of diligence and conflicts of interest.

I told Gary and Jeremy: "I can't in good conscience abandon my sole chance to make the doctors answer for what they had neglected to do. The doctors must be included in the lawsuit."

That would limit us to an individual action. I was hoping Jeremy and Gary would agree to represent us on a contingency basis either way. Both lawyers knew I wanted to win a substantial claim against Johnson & Johnson in Vanessa's name. But we'd have to win significant punitive damages to cover more than the legal costs, something that would be very hard to do.

I remember the silence in the room. They thought I had lost it. A guy who could end up losing his house. I understood that. I certainly wasn't in a very strong bargaining position. I was offering them no money upfront, an iffy case against three very powerful organizations who never give up, and insisting we do it the hard way. The only thing I really had on my side was the truth. Would it be enough?

Gary didn't back down. He wanted to protect me against making a decision I might regret. But we were out of time. He suggested a compromise to keep my options open: we would file two lawsuits at the same time. Jeremy agreed, although he did not appear to be happy as we parted.

On September 18, 2000, we filed a class action for $100 million with the Superior Court of Justice in Toronto against Johnson & Johnson, Janssen-Ortho Inc., McNeil Consumer Products and Health Canada. Vanessa was the representative plaintiff. We sent out a media release to help get the word out to attract calls from more victims.

We also filed an individual action for $11 million discreetly in the Milton courthouse, just twenty-five minutes north of Oakville. We claimed against Janssen-Ortho Inc., Johnson & Johnson, Health Canada, the Ontario College of Pharmacists, the pharmacy that sold us Prepulsid and the four doctors that treated Vanessa.[2] The suits were filed, but not served to the defendants. They still hadn't seen them. We would wait until after the inquest to decide which suit to serve to the defendants.

As I drove home that day I knew Gloria and I had just begun the battle of our lives. The odds were stacked against us. But I had a chance to expose so many unhealthy practices in the pharmaceutical industry. If I didn't, who would? As a member of provincial parliament I was known for my stubborn streak and had a reputation for speaking my mind. If I backed down, how could anyone without my experience stand a chance?

I continued my investigation, spending hundreds of hours researching long QT and Prepulsid. We had to convince the inquest jury of two things: First, there was nothing wrong with Vanessa's heart. Of course it is almost impossible to prove a negative. It would be easier for the other side—by planting seeds of doubt.

Second, we must prove that Prepulsid stopped Vanessa's heart. We had good evidence of this—and evidence that Health Canada knew the risks fifteen months before. But would the jury accept a normal standard of proof—what is "probable"[3]—or get mesmerized by expert testimony about "cause and effect." If they fell into the "cause and effect" trap, I thought we could lose.

Sana Sukkari explained why: cause and effect is a higher standard of proof than any court in the world. Instead of "beyond a reasonable doubt," like in a criminal court, it means virtually certain. I was surprised to hear that cigarettes have never been proven to cause lung cancer by "cause and effect." Yet everyone knows long-term smoking causes lung cancer. That's how tough the standard is to prove.

To prove a drug can stop a patient's heart by cause and effect a researcher would have to go through a three-step process: give a drug to a patient and record the deadly heart arrhythmia. Then withdraw the drug, and record the arrhythmia going away. And then give them the drug again—*and record the exact same reaction*. That would be foolish and unethical. No researcher would complete step three—stopping a patient's heart a second time—because it's too dangerous. Step three simply can't be completed for serious adverse reactions. So instead, the drug companies just put the drugs on the market. And when the body count begins, they point out subtle differences with each deceased patient: the dose must have been *too high*; "at a lower dose our drug would not be the cause." *Another drug* the patient was taking interfered; "our drug alone was not the cause." The patient was old and *couldn't metabolize* the drug; "our drug does not cause that in younger patients." The patient *had a condition* that interfered with the drug; "our drug was not the cause." And so on. Drug labels keep getting longer, sales keep growing, and no one tells our doctors.

We also might have to deal with: "The patient had a previously unknown and hidden heart condition that by coincidence mimics the adverse reaction our drug is known for"—even if there was no evidence of one.

I felt sure that's what they were going to try to do to Vanessa. Gloria and I had monitored Vanessa's health very closely. One of us had taken Vanessa to each and every doctor's appointment. She was healthy girl who weighed 140 pounds. She was athletic, graceful, and glowed with health. She had an off-and-on stomach problem common to teenage girls—throwing up after meals—but had it under control. Was it bulimia? Dr. Kayner felt she had a mild form of bulimia. But never in her life before she took Prepulsid had she even fainted. There was absolutely nothing wrong with her heart.

Gary warned me that if some scientist with a lot of letters after his name got on the stand and used medical-speak in front of a jury the outcome could be surprising. Juries tended to trust experts, even if they'd never seen the patient. So in an abundance of caution Madeline and Hart had to have their hearts checked to see if they had so-called congenital long QT. Somehow I knew they were both normal. And that's the way their tests turned out. We also checked on both sides of our family way back for any history of heart arrhythmia. There was none. There was simply no substance to any potential theory that Vanessa had a faulty heart. But I was still very uneasy.

Then things took a somewhat eerie turn. I received a letter from the coroner providing details of the inquest. The inquest would be held at the John Sopinka Courthouse in Hamilton, beginning on March 19, 2001, exactly one year after Vanessa had died. During my investigation of Vanessa's death, one of the things I'd discovered was that if I dug deep enough, I could find a reason for everything that had happened. I'd really stopped believing in coincidences. Nothing happens by accident. So I couldn't help wondering what significance there was in that date being chosen—the saddest date in our lives. Was someone watching out for us? Was this a good omen, or bad?

As my binder with articles and clinical studies on Prepulsid grew bigger I had started to feel like a criminal investigator. I knew the antihistamine Seldane had been pulled off the market in 1998 after patients died of heart arrhythmias.[4] Had other drugs as well? Outside of the world's most infamous drug disaster—thalidomide—it was extremely difficult to find information on drugs that had been taken off the market. It was like they'd never existed. I spent a lot of time in libraries and on the Internet researching drug names in old periodicals, and found reference to the drug Dr. Joel Lexchin had mentioned—Zomax, a Johnson & Johnson painkiller.

The similarities between Prepulsid and painkiller Zomax were uncanny. Zomax caused deadly anaphylactic reactions. The label changes had proven ineffective, more deadly adverse reactions occurred, and finally it was withdrawn. Eventually, 187 reported deaths had been reported related to Zomax.

Late one night I stumbled across a revealing article on the Internet from December 1991 in *The Washington Monthly*, by Morton Mintz. It told the story of Suprol (suprofen) marketed by another Johnson & Johnson subsidiary McNeil. In one clinical study before FDA approval nine out of twenty-four young male volunteers suffered mild or moderate flank pain. Three others had signs of renal (kidney) toxicity. Nevertheless Suprol was approved for sale in December 1985, and in April 1986 McNeil sent out the first of three "Dear Doctor" letters about reports of "abrupt flank pain." By June the FDA had ninety reports of kidney damage and ordered McNeil to send another "Dear Doctor" letter. By October, Johnson & Johnson's U.K. subsidiary pulled Suprol off the U.K. market "on commercial grounds," *but in the U.S. McNeil just sent out a third "Dear Doctor" letter*. This sounded so familiar to me. Finally on May 13, 1997, European authorities recommended the complete withdrawal of Suprol. Two days later McNeil gave up and pulled Suprol in the U.S. More than three hundred cases of flank pain had been reported as well as those with kidney damage.

There also appeared to me an alarming historical pattern with Johnson & Johnson drugs: arrhythmias. Clinium (lidoflazine) was pulled off the market in 1989, and Hismanal (astemizole) in 1999 related to arrhythmias. Risperidal (risperidone), Haldol (haloperidol) and Motilium could also cause long QT, and a group of drugs that ended in ". . . azole" (some of them from other drug companies)—when combined with other drugs. Vascor (bepridil) was taken off the market later.

It seemed that Johnson & Johnson drug developers must have a lot of experience with drugs that could cause long QT. It was almost like they specialized in them. Why would a company do that? I got a possible answer when I spoke to Dr. Ray Woosley at Georgetown University, the leading expert on long QT and unofficial keeper of the list of drugs that can cause long

QT.⁵ Ray was also highly motivated to reduce adverse reactions, as his own brother died after taking Prepulsid. He was dedicated to educating others about long QT. I gazed out the window of my ground floor office on a sunny September afternoon as Ray educated me by long distance.

"Why was Prepulsid still available?" I asked Ray. "It had over forty contraindications."

"The FDA was disappointed with the Prepulsid labeling— the label clutter. Instead of withdrawing the drug, the company adjusted the label, knowing no one reads it."

"What about SIDS?" I asked. "Six-month-old Gage Stevens' death had originally had been blamed on that."

"It's quite possible other SIDS deaths were caused by Prepulsid," he said. "Some with erythromycin, and some on its own." To this day I don't know if SIDS researchers have made that connection.

"Why don't doctors do a better job of warning patients about adverse drug reactions?"

There was a long pause.

"Medical schools don't teach about drug toxicity," he said at last. "There are few courses in pharmacology [how drugs work in the body] in medical schools. Drug education is basically left up to the drug companies. Many cardiologists [heart specialists] don't even know what torsades de pointes is. Only two pediatric pharmacologists graduated in the entire U.S. last year; and twenty adult pharmacologists."

Not even one per state.

"Prepulsid was on the Canadian market for ten years," I said. "How could no one have noticed the true risks?" Despite losing a brother who died while on Prepulsid, Ray was very professional and fair-minded.

"People at drug companies are honest, but they make mistakes. They get paid to develop good news on one drug type.

Bad news could lose them their jobs. They don't look for toxicity data. When the FDA first uncovered the Seldane problem, they went through their files and discovered twenty other ADR cases in their own files. They were there. Just no one had read the adverse reports."

"But the drug companies must keep their own records of adverse reactions."

"MacNeil (Johnson & Johnson) had ongoing problems with their 'azole' group," he said. "They all have a similar structure. But no one was looking for these reactions in the eighties. The problem is the subsidiaries don't talk to each other. They work on different metabolites (molecules made from an original molecule). And there is no corporate memory."

With the greatest respect for Ray, at this point I'd learned too much to believe the problem was lack of "corporate memory." Johnson & Johnson had owned MacNeil Labs, Ortho Pharmaceutical and Janssen Pharmaceutica. I could not believe that Johnson & Johnson executives had not asked a lot of questions about why a number of their drugs that caused long QT and heart arrhythmias had to be taken off the market. I felt quite sure they would remember these things.

Ray referred me to Dr. Jack Utrecht M.D., Ph.D, a professor of Pharmacy and Medicine at the University of Toronto—a leading Canadian authority on adverse drug reactions. He chaired the Medical Research Council of Canada Grants Committee for Pharmaceutical Sciences from 1992 to 1997, and in 2001 was awarded the Canada Research Chair in Adverse Drug Reactions and chaired the Health Canada Scientific Advisory Panel on Hepatotoxicity. His research is focused on the mechanisms of idiosyncratic drug reactions. Jack was a big help to me over five years and we met several times after my first call.

"The problem with cisapride was known a year ago, long

before March 2000." he said candidly. "But once a doctor finds a drug reliable, they simply trust it."

"It was vague," I said. "But there was information available to doctors on the risks of Prepulsid elsewhere."

"Doctors don't read the Adverse Drug Reaction Newsletter. The CPS (*Compendium of Pharmaceuticals and Specialties*) is there to protect the pharmaceutical companies. Few doctors read it." This was the third expert who told me most doctors simply don't read about adverse reactions.

"Why didn't Johnson & Johnson pull Prepulsid off the market sooner?"

Jack's answer was illuminating.

"A drug becomes a child to the developer. When it is withdrawn it is hard on the researcher. They hate to see it die."

I later learned that Dr. Paul Janssen, the founder and lead researcher at Janssen Pharmaceutica in Belgium, was a brilliant scientist who personally held a hundred patents for prescription drugs. I discovered a lengthy interview with him on the Internet where he described manipulating or "tweaking" chemical structures (molecules) to predict their biological effects on the body to create new drugs.[6] But Paul had a reputation for being aggressive, and for pushing things. One researcher I interviewed described him as an "autocrat who made things happen," so I was not surprised to read Paul's comments on adverse reactions: "When chloroform was killing 1 per cent of patients this was, I wouldn't say accepted—it was certainly regretted—but it didn't stop physicians from using chloroform, and I never heard of legal consequences when somebody was killed by it. Today for the slightest thing going wrong patients go and see a lawyer."

I found this comment chilling. First, because "regretted" is a not a word most people would use to describe the death of human being. And he'd almost said "accepted." Second, using chloroform to facilitate lifesaving surgery was a far cry from using a drug like Prepulsid for bloating. And third, I didn't believe patients would go and see a lawyer for the slightest thing going wrong. In fact, with over 2 million serious adverse drug reactions a year in the U.S., and a possible 200,000 deaths, I believe the opposite was true. Most patients don't even know what happened to them. I don't want to say I found Dr. Janssen uncaring, but I certainly didn't want anyone like him on our jury.

"How could we reduce adverse drug reactions?" I asked Jack.

"Well, Accutane can cause worse birth defects than thalidomide, and they sell it to young women for acne. But it requires written consent. The patient signs a form. That helps."

That was the first I'd heard of written consent for a prescription drug—like surgery. If every patient had to sign their name when getting a prescription, it would require that the doctor learn the risks, and explain them.

"Although it wouldn't always work," Jack continued. "There might be three thousand patients who take the drug in Phase III of testing—the last phase before approval. A very rare serious adverse reaction might only affect one in ten thousand patients, and will only show up in Phase IV of testing—the open market."

If you take any new drug, even free samples, you are joining a giant drug trial, becoming part of a giant Big Pharma experiment—Phase IV of testing. Doctors never tell patients that. Rare and very rare dangers aren't recognized until tens of thousands of patients take the drug. A lot of injuries can occur before a bad drug is withdrawn. Here's the math: if one in ten thousand people will suffer liver damage from a new drug—and a million people take the new drug, that's a hundred people who will need a new liver, or die.

If you have ever bought a major lottery ticket like 6/49, your odds of winning were about 1 in 14 million. But you could only lose $2. If you take a new drug on the market that turns out to have a dangerous side effect, your odds of losing could be 1 in 10,000—1,400 times greater. But you are betting your life. Taking a new drug is your lottery ticket.

And even with written and informed consent, the adverse reaction warning must be comprehensive. The Accutane patient consent form each female patient must sign before getting the drug warned clearly about the risk of birth defects, but was not given to males. I discovered later that week I wasn't the only politician who lost a child to a prescription drug. Bart Stupak Jr. the seventeen-year-old son of Congressman Bart Stupak of Michigan had committed suicide after taking Accutane for several months on May 14, 2000. Bart's parents were shocked to find out that the FDA Medwatch had published a warning from Roche Laboratories in a "Dear Doctor" letter on February 1998, twenty-seven months earlier: *Accutane may cause depression, psychosis and, rarely, suicidal ideation, suicide attempts and suicide.*[7] Two weeks before the FDA had approved a new label for Accutane which added *emotional instability* and *depression* to the warnings.

More drug warnings never received.

"Doctors see an awful lot of adverse drug reactions. Why don't they report them more often?" I asked Jack.

"Serious reactions are rare. It's extremely difficult to get a reliable reporting system, and to know when one has happened. If reports are incomplete or inaccurate they are useless. There's another reason. The information on adverse reactions does not get dealt with in any useful way by Health Canada."

I was to learn Jack was right about Health Canada. In fairness to doctors, no one at Health Canada does much with the reports. This was proven true in August 2004 when the federal government put $187.5 million into approving drugs faster, instead of tracking adverse reactions—from everything I'd learned, the exact opposite of what they should have done.[8] The Health Canada group that monitored drugs on the market got only $2.5 million and actually *gave up assigning and tracking the cause of adverse drug reactions.*[9] They actually accept the reports and don't investigate the "why." That's like the police finding someone injured or dead on the street and just writing a report.

This wasn't entirely new. Dr. Joel Lexchin later showed that since 1960 forty-one drugs had been pulled off the market in Canada, but no one at Health Canada had kept comprehensive record of why.[10] This explains a lot. Philosopher George Santayana said, "Those who cannot remember the past are doomed to repeat it." The $60 million the government spent to get answers on Swiss Air Flight 111 would help prevent similar disasters. But if no one in Canada tracked why drug disasters happened, why wouldn't they continue?

FRIDAY OCTOBER 6, 2000, was our worst day since Vanessa's funeral.

Jeremy Taylor had called me from the highway two days before. I'd spent many hours doing research with the bright co-op student Jeremy had hired. Our agreement appeared to be working well. But Gary Will's associate, Chris Morrison, had told Jeremy that it was problematic to have Vanessa act as representative plaintiff in the class action, while at the same time maintaining that her death was due to the negligence of the doctors. This meant I might not be able to lead a class action.

Jeremy's tone was a lot different than before. He told me his two Oakville partners were concerned with the time he'd spent on the case, and that I owed him $30,000 to date. I was shocked. This was right out of the blue. Our agreement was on contingency only. He had never asked me for a cent up front before. He also said if the class action was never certified I might have to cover the legal costs. Another surprise. I'd thought of Jeremy as a good friend. Yet he was behaving as if our agreement didn't exist.

"I'll be in the office on Friday afternoon," he told me.

And he was. His mood hadn't changed. "I need you to give me six thousand dollars and a thousand dollars a month," he demanded. I'd been selling RRSPs until my business built up, which is why I'd accepted the deal he offered weeks before. I told him I didn't have the money.

"You have *money*. You bought a new van and took your family to Florida."

I was mortified. "I leased the van and the trip was a gift," I clarified for him.

He railed at me, "Look, you've got to make a decision. I can't keep financing this case forever. You think you're going to get a million dollars. You're not."

We had never even discussed any such amount. Clearly Jeremy was under some urgent financial pressure and needed a guarantee of some payment as we moved forward. But what did his behaviour say about our chances of winning? Was our case still good? Had he learned something he wasn't telling me? And I'd never heard of a class action where the plaintiffs pay the lawyers until it is certified. This was surreal.

Everything was falling apart. My face was flushed and my heart pounded. I struggled for what to say, "I'll have to get independent legal advice."

"Then you're no longer my client," he announced angrily and walked out.

I'd just been fired by my lawyer. The man I'd trusted. I dreaded so much telling Gloria what happened. She would be devastated. One thing I knew for sure: I had to get out my office—out of his building.

I stopped at a truck rental place on the way home. By 2 p.m. the next day—Saturday—I was totally out, not even a paper clip left on the carpet. Everything from my office was in our recreation room, my new office. Things got worse before they got better. Jeremy also refused to give me two boxes of evidence and research materials we'd assembled over months until I agreed to pay him six thousand dollars. This was hard on me, but worse for Gloria. The last thing we needed was another battle. Especially with someone we'd thought of as a friend. I told her that I thought Gary Will would still take our case without Jeremy's involvement. That was bravado. I wasn't so sure.

The following week I drove to Toronto, took the elevator up to the 30th floor of the Simpson's Tower on Bay Street, and waited in the windowed boardroom of Will Barristers LLP for Gary Will. Gazing out at the grey clouds over the Toronto islands and Lake Ontario, I knew I was in deep trouble. If Jeremy wanted out, how long would it be before Gary did the same? This was a very tough case. And I was going backwards. The legal costs for the inquest—which might take weeks—would be in the tens of thousands of dollars. I was in no position to pay one lawyer, let alone two. As I sat in the silence of that boardroom I began to think irrationally, foolishly—wondering if I could tackle the inquest on my own, question all the witnesses, persuade the jury.

Then Gary came in, mild-mannered and pleasant as usual. I described to him in detail what had happened with Jeremy.

"Let me talk with Jeremy about getting the two boxes of evidence," he said calmly. "His situation is different from mine. I can take your case without any payment from you before its conclusion. The most important thing is that the opposition don't think that part of your legal team has lost faith in your case or abandoned the claim."

I was dumbfounded. It took a few seconds to sink in. Gary

was sticking with us. And Vanessa.

An hour later I was in my car heading back to Oakville on the QEW, with good news for Gloria. We were on.

Gary Will was our lifeline in those days.

The following week film maker Erna Buffie called. Health Canada had refused to give her key documents she'd requested, like the 1990 new drug application for Prepulsid. "They said it was proprietary information that belonged to Johnson & Johnson," she explained. "How can safety information be a commercial secret?"

Good question. The information that drug companies give our regulators to get their drugs approved is simply not available. So the terrific researchers like Joel Lexchin who are focused on safety can't look for evidence of risk in their early trials.

Yet we were to learn that keeping new drug applications secret is normal at Health Canada, and Erna had to hire specialists in using the Freedom of Information (FOI) process to get the documents. In the U.S. they are made available on the Internet for the same drugs! Every public statement Health Canada officials made was about how concerned they were with safety, and every action they took blocked our progress. I no longer had any doubt that Health Canada was Big Pharma's partner.

Meanwhile phone calls to me from people who said they had suffered injuries from Prepulsid kept coming. I listened to them all, offered help where I could, and took notes. One afternoon I received a call in my new home office from a woman in British Columbia. She was weeping as she began telling me her story, something I was getting used to—another person who had lost a loved one. I sat back listening intently.

The lady was talking about Prepulsid alright. But it wasn't a family member that had died that she wept over. It was her dog. She been feeding Prepulsid to him for spitting up and he died suddenly. I was shaken. I had no clue they gave the same drugs to animals as humans—and for similar symptoms. The whole idea made me feel nauseous. This lady was obviously grieving, but I admit it was hard to listen to.

When I hung up the phone I searched on the Internet and it was all there. Veterinarians gave the stuff to cats and dogs, horses, and even elephants. The animals suffered some of the same adverse reactions as humans. This lady's dog on Prepulsid had died suddenly like Vanessa. It made me realize that Big Pharma isn't in the drug business for people. They are in the drug business for mammals—all Big Pharma customers. How many mammals had died after taking Prepulsid? I wondered. I was sure a jury would want to know the answer. How sad. This call pushed me over the edge. I wept as well. God, I missed Vanessa.

Chapter 12

Games with Names

*"From antiquity, people have recognized the connection
between naming and power."*
—Casey Miller and Kate Swift

*"Speak English!" said the Eaglet. "I don't know the meaning
of half those long words, and I don't believe you do either."*
—Lewis Carroll, *Alice's Adventures in Wonderland*

November 2000

GETTING A DRUG NAME WRONG could cost a human life. It
happens all the time. Canada and the world could have learned
critical lessons from the thalidomide disaster in the early
1960s—if they had paid attention. Thalidomide (a generic
name) originated in Germany and was sold in the late 1950s and
early 1960s over the counter as a sleeping pill, and to help pregnant women deal with morning sickness. It was sold in forty-
six countries, but had more than fifty brand names.[1] As many as
four thousand infants died at birth and another eight thousand

survived with severe internal injuries or deformities because their mothers took thalidomide during pregnancy.

Two vital lessons from thalidomide have been ignored by drug companies and regulators. While unborn infants were being injured, Canada, Japan, and Italy delayed taking thalidomide off the market for months after most of Europe did. When reading the horror stories from Europe about a drug called Contergan, regulators and doctors elsewhere had no reason to relate it to Neurosedyn in Sweden, Distival in Britain, or Verdil in Brazil[2]—three other names for thalidomide.

Brand names for prescription drugs should have been abolished after thalidomide. They exist for marketing purposes and confuse doctors and regulators who need to know the true risks of drugs. Brand names are a key way that Big Pharma confuses patients and manipulates our emotions to sell their drugs.

The second lesson was that communication between regulatory agencies needed to improve. This is still a major problem. Journalists have been key in exposing unsafe drugs—from thalidomide to today.[3] And cisapride is still sold in many countries. But it is difficult for investigators or patients to spot trouble because of the many names under which cisapride is sold. I spent hundreds of hours searching for information on Prepulsid from across the world. I would Google Prepulsid and get Canadian stories, but miss U.S. stories because Prepulsid is spelled with an "o" in the U.S.—Propulsid. I got more hits using the generic name "cisapride." And then one day a list of brand names for cisapride worldwide popped up on my screen. It stopped me cold. I found a total of twenty-nine different names. I tried to imagine the hundreds of media stories I had missed worldwide that might have used these brand names. Just like a mother in India, worried about her child might easily miss reading the story of a fifteen-year-old-girl in Ontario, Canada, who died from Prepulsid, because she is searching under the names Cisawal, Esorid, or Guptro.[4]

It's helpful to look at how a drug gets to us.

Do you remember the periodic chart of the elements on the wall in grade ten science class? Oxygen was O. Hydrogen was H. Potassium was K, and so on. A simple basic molecule is water (H_2O), two atoms of hydrogen and one of oxygen bound together. Well, prescription drugs are bigger, more complex molecules, with a number of elements put together in a unique way.

Researchers create new drugs in labs by modifying molecules. Drug companies and governments pay researchers to do that in private labs and at our universities. Each new molecule may end up as a new drug, also called a new chemical entity (NCE) or compound. If after some initial testing it looks promising, they seek a potentially lucrative patent. The drug companies tell us that only about one in ten thousand new compounds reach the market. Promising compounds are tested first on animals, and then the company seeks permission to start human testing. In the U.S. this is called an investigational new drug application (IND). Their goal is a new drug application (NDA) and approval. That requires highly regulated testing of the compound on humans, first on healthy humans, and at a later stage on people with the condition or disease being treated. But this part of the drug development cycle can take two to eight years or longer, a source of great frustration for Big Pharma. Because during that time, their exclusive twenty-year patent is running out. Once approved, a year's exclusive sales could mean billions in sales—millions of dollars a day. So time is money.

Human testing is done in four phases.

Phase I is usually done on twenty to eighty healthy young adult males who are paid, looking mostly at safety: what the drug does to their bodies, and at what dose it either works, or intolerable side effects appear. This is risky. For example, in March 2006 six young men were rushed to hospital in London,

England, with multiple organ failure after participating in such a trial for an experimental drug.

Phase II is usually twenty to three hundred volunteers some of whom have the condition being addressed, looking mostly to see if the drug works on the targeted symptoms, but also toxicity.

In Phase III the drug is administered to three hundred to three thousand patients, most of whom have the condition being targeted and who might be on other drugs (in a randomized-controlled way). Some subjects get the drug, others will get a placebo.

If after Phase III the drug appears to be safe and effective, all the documentation is compiled into a new drug application (NDA), usually delivered to the FDA and Health Canada in numerous boxes filling one or more large trucks. Then some lucky doctor/drug reviewer is assigned the responsibility to pore over all these documents and say yes or no; they can sell it for that condition, or they can't.

But Phase IV is the drug being sold to the public. This is where children, pregnant women, millions of people on other drugs, and anyone taking the drug for a longer term become canaries in a mine for Big Pharma. No one knows what will happen. That's why doctors like David Knox and the people at Public Citizen suggest you stay away from new drugs for at least seven years.

All drugs have three names: a chemical name, a generic name, and a brand name—which is trademarked by the drug company (owned and protected by law).[5] Each name is regulated under different rules. So if you get confused, you are in good company. According to the *Journal of the American Pharmacists Association*[6] there are more than nine thousand generic drug names, and 33,000 trademarked brand names in use in the U.S. That number may be smaller in Canada. But it is obviously far too many names for any doctor or pharmacist to remember.

The chemical name is used only by researchers. Patients never see it.

At the end of twenty years in Canada and the U.S. brand-name drugs go "off-patent." That means any manufacturer can create an exact copy of the molecule and sell the drug under its generic or drug name. Of course they must meet high-quality standards. There is a huge secondary business worldwide referred to as the generic industry. Generic drugs usually cost much less than brand drugs cost—perhaps 50 to 70 per cent. The public gets a break on brand prices after twenty years. It's supposed to be simple. But disagreements between the brand companies and the generic companies are the source of innumerable lawsuits back and forth costing hundreds of millions of dollars. Patients pay for these costs when they buy drugs.

The generic name is not proprietary, meaning there is no trademark or ownership of the name. It identifies a unique molecule (compound) and is used by doctors, pharmacists and scientists worldwide, which is why it's also known as the common name, or drug name. Prepulsid's generic name is cisapride.

The World Health Organization has to approve each common name for new drugs. Common names are usually longer than brand names, are written without capitals (like cisapride), and are created when a drug is ready for market. A U.S. government body called the United States Adopted Names Council (USANC) selects the generic names. They try to help ensure safety, consistency, and logic in names to avoid confusion, which can be dangerous. So they use certain groups of letters (stems) as a clue to doctors about what kind of drug it is—the drug class. Stems can appear as prefixes, infixes, or suffixes. A generic drug names get longer, they are increasingly difficult to spell, pronounce, and remember—the ultimate medical-speak.

If the stem "adol" appears in the drug name, like tazadolene, the drug is an analgesic. If the name ends with "ac," like

Bromfenac, it's an anti-inflammatory drug. The suffix "coxib," like the arthritis drugs celecoxib (Celebrex), valdecoxib (Bextra), and rofecoxib (Vioxx), identifies the class of COX-2 inhibitors. They all help reduce pain in a certain way. The last five letters will provide a clue to your doctor about how the drug works. And since similar drugs can cause similar side effects, if your doctor is up to date he should caution you about what adverse effects to watch for. Many don't.

Some people feel that since Vioxx was pulled off the market for causing over one hundred thousand heart attacks and strokes, a caution should be issued in this whole class of drugs. Vioxx (rofecoxib) and Bextra (valdecoxib) have now both been taken off the market for similar reasons. And at least one study I found suggests Celebrex may cause similar problems.[7] According to Public Citizen's *Worst Pills, Best Pills*, two older painkillers for arthritis in a different class of drugs (NSAIDS) appear to be safer: Tylenol (acetaminophen) and Motrin (ibuprofen), although no drug is completely safe. Without Public Citizen, most patients would have almost no way to know which drug might be taken off the market next.

There is a problem you may have noticed: generic names often sound or look very much alike, which can contribute to medication errors. Doctors are human; they might forget if the drug they think will help you is celecoxib or rofecoxib, or might confuse Prednisolone (Prelone) with prednisone (Deltasone)— both adrenal steroids used for asthma and other conditions. The people at USANC try to assign generic names that are easy to say. Obviously they are running out of short names. Most new generic names have four syllables. Medication errors will increase unless they adopt better ways to identify generic drugs.

Brand names—like Vioxx—are capitalized, just like a person's name, and are the names you see in drug ads. They are protected by trademark law, like Ford Focus or Coke, and approved in Canada as part of market authorization by Health Canada. The drug company owns the right to the name by trademark and they protect it. In a world where a new drug could be worth billions in profits, drug companies live or die by their trademarked brand names. If anyone gets too close to copying their brand names, they'll end up in court.

Some drugs are actually natural compounds found in nature. In fact, of 520 new pharmaceutical products approved in the UK between 1983 and 1994, about four out of ten were actually natural products or made from natural products. And "60 to 80 per cent of lifesaving antibacterials and anti-cancer drugs were derived from natural products."[8] Aspirin is really acetylsalicylic acid—very similar to methyl salicylate, found in the bark of the willow tree. Our First Nations people discovered centuries ago that tea made from willow tree bark reduced fever and pain. But no company owns the exclusive rights or patent to sell aspirin.

Drug patents give one company the exclusive rights to make and sell a molecule (drug) for a period of time—in Canada it's twenty years. That's how Big Pharma makes money. With the hope of finding lifesaving drugs, or at least finding drugs that effectively treat symptoms, governments award patents even on products drawn from nature. It costs a lot of money to conduct research. By awarding exclusive marketing rights for a period of time to a molecule or compound, governments create a legal right to get that investment back, and then make a return or profit on it. How much profit on a monopoly product is in the public interest? Is 12 per cent return for shareholders fair, or is a retirement package worth $190 million for a CEO necessary? Brand names are normally created far in advance of the drug getting on the market, even before testing on humans. After testing on animals, they have a hopeful idea of at least one medicinal effect it will likely have on a human body, and have studied the potential market carefully. In other words they know what they want to sell it for, and likely how much money they want to make. But sometimes the names are registered first, long before the companies even have a drug for the name. They just like the sound of it. Brand names are so important that Big Pharma is also referred to as the brand companies. And the brand companies will pay up to a million dollars to naming consultants to come up with a cool new brand name that attracts consumers (all paid for by you in the price of the drugs you buy).

But there is a basic conflict. Consumers like to see some indication of what a drug does in its name. But no brand name is supposed to make or imply a medical claim or promise. So we'll never see a prescription drug named Nopain or Cancerpause. Rogaine, sold to help grow hair, was supposed to be Regain,[9] but the FDA turned down the name Regain. It sounds like a promise.

Neither are names allowed which suggest a use for which the drug is not approved. So Zoloft, sold to treat depression and never approved for children would not have been allowed to be named anything like Childpax or Teenium. Eprex has been used off-label by high-altitude cycling competitors in Europe in a risky attempt to get more oxygen to their muscles. Regulators would never have approved names like Speedex or Prorace for this drug.

Big Pharma does not choose brand names to help improve patient safety. Naming strategies are based on subtle but powerful marketing tricks to get you and your doctor attracted and hooked subconsciously. And they work. Why else would anyone pay a million dollars to develop a name? The problem is that names can subconsciously exaggerate benefits, skewing risk/benefit ratios and undermining what drug safety is all about.

Let me show you what I mean. Eli Lilly's Serafem, marketed for women with PMDD (bad periods) sounds like seraphim,

which means angel.[10] The "phim" is replaced with "fem"—
short for feminine. A feminine angel. Doesn't that sound nice?
Especially when you hear how the Serafem label describes
PMDD symptoms: "irritability, mood swings and tension." It
also says these symptoms can "cause interference in day-to-day
activities and relationships."

Who wouldn't rather be a feminine angel?

But watch out: Serafem is actually Prozac (fluoxetine
hydrochloride)—a drug that has a battered reputation and
brand due to widely reported side effects being masked with a
new name. Surprise. So patients prescribed Serafem have lost
their best chance of being alerted to the risks of the medicine
they are given—the name—and if, like many people, they have
partially consumed prescriptions left over in their medicine
cabinet, they could conceivably end up taking Serafem and
Prozac at the same time, causing a dangerous overdose.

Any patient who bothered to read the approved U.S. Prozac
label would find *twenty-nine pages* of small print. Next time
you are at your computer Google "Prozac official prescribing
information" and take a look. You'll see that Prozac might
infrequently or rarely cause patients over two hundred and forty
adverse effects including rash, anorexia, and convulsions. And
that more than one out of ten patients taking Prozac in trials
suffered from anxiety, nervousness, or insomnia. Prozac taken
with thioridazine could possibly cause death from arrhythmia,
the same way Vanessa died.[11] The FDA has issued two special
warnings about increased risk of suicide with Prozac. The latest
warning, in July 2005, reads that antidepressants like Prozac
"may increase suicidal thoughts and actions in about one out of
fifty people eighteen years or younger."

The Sarafem label on the other hand is only twenty-three
pages long. Since dosages vary anyway, what important safety
information might have been omitted that was on the other six

pages of the Prozac label? In case doctors and patients aren't completely confused in trying to find out if Prozac is safe for them or not, here's the first sentence on the U.S. Prozac label under Clinical Pharmacology: "The antidepressant actions of fluoxetine are presumed to be linked to its inhibition of CNS neuronal uptake of serotonin."

The U.S. Serafem label reads: "The mechanism of action of fluoxetine in premenstrual dysphoric disorder (PMDD) is unknown, but it is presumed to be linked to its inhibition of CNS neuronal uptake of serotonin."

Presumed to be? Unknown?

In other words, no one is even sure how the stuff works! To prove an adverse drug reaction has occurred and help keep patients safe, the drug industry and our regulators insist on proof by "cause and effect." But to sell a blockbuster with proven risks, *presuming* what it does to the human brain is just fine.

And they've been selling it since the eighties. But you know what? People buy it. And they have nice new name for it that probably cost them a lot of money, so by God they're going to sell it—millions worth.

What's in a name? Money of course.

Here are a few more naming strategies I uncovered that Big Pharma uses to get inside your head: "Lipid regulator" is shortened into Lipitor by joining the words and removing seven letters in the middle. Lipitor lowers so-called "bad cholesterol" and is now the world's largest-selling drug—exceeding $14 billion in 2007. It has been known to cause a severe and painful muscle-wasting disease that can destroy a person's kidneys, and memory loss.

Viagra also comes from two words—vital and Niagara, or vigor and Niagara. What man who has erectile dysfunction doesn't want to be as vital or vigorous as the great Niagara Falls? Under certain conditions Viagra can cause side effects that of course are certainly not hinted in the name—death and blindness.

Levitra was designed to siphon away a portion of the millions in market share from Viagra. With Levitra, the naming specialists used a different trick to get around the rules. Take a look at the next two sentences and see if they make sense to you:

Can yuo udnrestsnd tihs? Rseaerchres at Cmabrigde Uinervitsy hvee shwne the haumn mnid redas the wrod as a wolhe, so the ordre of the letres is not ipmortant, if the fsrit and lsat leetrts are in the rghit palce.

The human mind reads the whole word, taking meaning from the jumbled letters. Levitra is a letter jumble from the word "elevate" by switching an "e" for an "r." Many male customers would subconsciously get this message without Bayer ever mentioning *what* they need to elevate. It's clever of course. But imagine if the drug companies put the same effort into safety as they do marketing. Here are few more examples of implied benefits in names:

Brand name	Sold to treat	Implication
Allegra	stuffy noses	Italian for "light and lively"
Paxil	depression/anxiety	Latin for "peace"—pax
Celebrex	pain	celebrate: party on dude
Valium	anxiety	Valley/Elysium (a heavenly valley)

Sometimes the drug companies choose a name that sounds like another drug for which their exclusive patent is running out. Since competitive generic companies can't use the brand name, that's when the brand investment really pays off, because brand names get "branded" in consumer's minds. They've seen it in their doctor's office on charts on the wall, on his coffee cup, in magazines, and in the middle of their favourite TV show. And most of all they've seen it in their medicine cabinet day after day. They trust that brand. They have taken it, sometimes for years and received a real or imagined benefit.

Schering's drug Clarinex, which was introduced to replace their $3-billion blockbuster Claritin is a good example. Both drugs are for runny noses. Claritin's patent ran out and consumers can now buy exact copies of Claritin for perhaps half the price from other companies as "loratadine." But Schering planned in advance. They had a new patent—Clarinex—lined up for their runny-nosed customers, a molecule and name very close to Claritin. Using heavy advertising they switched millions of their Claritin customers over to buy Clarinex, which had years of profitable patent protection ahead, paying almost twice what they had to for their runny-nose medication.

The safety issue is that the folks at Schering took the Claritin compound and "tweaked" it, creating a new drug. And the new drug may not work for all patients. But it will likely cause new adverse reactions, some of which may not show up for years. Claritin fans will pay a lot more money for a similar drug, with new risk. That is the essence the drug marketing. They get more money, and we get more risks.

The generic drug companies have a tough time overcoming brand loyalty, even for patients on fixed incomes who could pay a fraction of the price. And the brand companies do everything they can to make it as difficult as possible. Who's thinking about health care when all this is going on? Or safety?

Selling Power in a Name

Sometimes branding companies recommend names that use certain letters like "x" and "c" because they produce a harder tonality. They are appealing to the subconscious of consumers who want advanced and powerful drugs.[12] This might sound silly, but the letter "X" is associated with science fiction—the X-Men, *The X-files*, and high-tech stuff like XML, a computer language. It appears in the drug names Zyprexa, Nexium, Eprex, Effexor, Plavix, Celebrex and Fosamax, all triple blockbusters—seven of the twelve top-selling drugs worldwide in 2004. Patients in distress buy powerful drugs. This naming stuff works. But there will never be any hint of the power of adverse reactions in a drug name.

Sound-alike Names

Sometimes the brand names sound too similar to other drugs. And confusion can be deadly. A doctor must try to remember innumerable brand names and thousands of generic names accurately, and search his memory for any safety information he might have read or heard. Then he must write it down so your pharmacist can read it. Doctors' handwriting is no worse than anyone else's, but it's certainly more important. Where else does a human life depend on one person reading another's handwriting? Pharmacists not only have to read doctors' handwriting, but read hundreds of typed labels daily, often names with similar prefixes and suffixes. The outcomes can be deadly. In one example numerous errors occurred between Metadate, taken for attention deficit disorder, and methadone, including the death of eight-year-old boy.[13] In Canada, patients have died after being given the wrong cancer drug—vincristine, instead of vinblastine.[14]

In the U.S. modafinil is sold for narcolepsy and off-label for children with ADHD as Sparlon. How would American parents that travel know the drug that might rarely cause aggression, psychosis, and suicidal events is called Alertec in Canada, and Vigicer and Provigil elsewhere?[15]

The people at Big Pharma always claim safety is their prime objective. So what have they done since thalidomide to help investigators and the media identify serious adverse drug reactions related to a drug and quickly spread the word to reduce injuries and save lives? Here's a section from the black box warning for Lamictal (lamotrigine) which itself can cause severe rashes, including the life-threatening Stevens-Johnson syndrome. "Dispensing errors have occurred between Lamictal and other drugs, most commonly Lamisil, lamivudine, Ludiomil, labetalol, and Lomotil."

Confusion reigns.

By 2007 I'd found seventy-six different brand names for cisapride worldwide.

ON NOVEMBER 6, 2000, Health Canada issued a Public Advisory regarding phenylpropanolamine (PPA), a nasal decongestant in over sixty prescription and over-the-counter cold and allergy medications, because it was "associated" with hemorrhagic stroke. At first I had some hope that the fuss I'd been making had made a difference at Health Canada, as Jane Cooper had told me. Then I read that Health Canada was following the lead of the FDA, that had just recommended that consumers not use any products containing PPA. Maybe there was hope—this time the warnings had gone out on the same day.

Our first Christmas without Vanessa was six weeks away.

We have always been a family of faith, but I faced the coming holiday with great trepidation. Eight months is no time at all when you lose a child. Sometimes it felt like Vanessa had been gone eight days. At other times I could almost feel her presence. But every occasion that should have been joyful for us now had a flipside. Christmas in our family had been such an exciting and happy time. Now, when we were together we not only had to deal with our own grief, but each other's.

Grief times four.

Hart worked to adjust to grade nine at Oakville Trafalgar High School. Vanessa's friends there had befriended him. But he had a new identity now—he would always be seen as Vanessa's brother. He told me it constantly reminded him she wasn't there. Madeline was getting along in a totally new environment, making many new friends at Queen's University. We were grateful for that.

Gloria had gone back to work a week after Vanessa died, fundraising for St. Peter's Hospital. She was busy and successful, helping to organize their first golf tournament in October and their fundraising gala, coming later in November. The people there were very supportive. I didn't know it, however, but things were taking a quiet toll on her.

I was busy working for clients, and could channel my grief into my investigation. It was my way of continuing to be Vanessa's father. Some people might say I wasn't facing reality, avoiding my own grief—obsessed even. But I didn't care if our opponents at the coming inquest thought I was possessed—as long as it kept them guessing.

Sometimes I'd come home and tell my family what I'd discovered during that day to help our case. They'd feign interest, but I could tell it gave them no solace. They were being polite. I was trying to tie down every detail of our tragedy for the inquest, while they were trying to forget. It wasn't easy for any of us.

Part of Gloria's job for the hospital was meeting with potential donors, and one week she had meetings at several funeral homes in Hamilton. The following Saturday morning I came down to our laundry room to get a shirt and found her curled up in a fetal position against the clothes dryer, weeping uncontrollably. I tried my best to console her, but sometimes there is just so little to say. Gloria had been working steadily through the week, keeping up a brave front, and quietly grieving on weekends. I had to ask myself—was it selfish for me to continue along this road? I had a long way to go—years. My battle was going to get worse before it got better. How was it truly affecting Gloria, Madeline, and Hart? Was I really doing the right thing?

To this day I don't know. But I couldn't abandon Vanessa. I had made an oath. And if I didn't continue to act I was afraid the empty feeling would never, ever go away.

I did what I had to do.

We did get some practical help with our grief. Losing a child puts your world out of order. It's so hard to make any sense out of it. Sharon Pocock at Halton Family Services provided counselling that was very helpful to me and Gloria, especially her belief in not going through grief, but growing through it. Gloria had someone who understood. I learned a lot. Everyone grieves differently, and there are no time limits. If you have lost someone you love, especially a child, bereavement counselling can be a great help.

People in White Coats

Chapter 13

Do No Harm

"As to diseases, make a habit of two things—to help, or at least do no harm."
—Hippocrates, *The Epidemics*—fourth century B.C.E.

"The adventures first ... explanations take such a dreadful time."
—The Gryphon, *Alice's Adventures in Wonderland*, Lewis Carroll

DECEMBER WAS A STELLAR MONTH in my investigation. It appeared that Prepulsid had crept into the consciousness of journalists across North America. Maybe it was because children had died, I couldn't be sure, but this story had a life of its own. I picked up my phone one weekday afternoon and film maker Erna Buffie was on the other end. She was wound up.

"By 1998 Johnson & Johnson knew Prepulsid could be dangerous with electrolyte disorders—low potassium and magnesium—and had added reference to that on the label."

I told Erna I had known that. A condition of low electrolytes might have combined with Prepulsid to stop Vanessa's heart.

"But, gastroparesis often causes vomiting, which can *lead* to electrolyte disorders." The impact of this fact struck me immediately. If vomiting was a common result of gastroparesis, Prepulsid should have been contraindicated for treating gastroparesis.

Erna continued: "And the most common side effect of Prepulsid, diarrhea, *also* causes electrolyte disorders. Over 14 per cent of people taking Prepulsid in testing—one out of seven—had diarrhea. So Prepulsid might cause heart arrhythmia not only with a common symptom of what it treated, but *also with its own most common side effect!* It should have definitely been taken off the market by the latest in 1998."

Erna had also finally obtained the documents through the Freedom of Information Act (FOI) that Health Canada had previously refused to release, including copies of all the emails that had gone back and forth between Health Canada official Marta Caris and Janssen officials in February 2000, when the final Prepulsid warning letter was being delayed, the fateful last warning Dr. Kayner never saw.

"Janssen didn't fax the final warning letter until Health Canada basically threatened to send it out to the doctors themselves," she said.

She also had a copy of Health Canada's report on their internal investigation into Prepulsid *after* Vanessa died, dated April 17, 2000. There was sorrow in her voice as she read me the conclusion: "The efficacy of cisapride relative to placebo appears to be modest and inconsistent . . . the risk associated with cisapride does not appear to justify its continued use . . ." and added, "They finally took it off the market because it hardly worked."

I closed my eyes and took a deep breath, feeling the sorrow as well. Then I exhaled, feeling a familiar ache in my head.

Nevertheless, I felt Erna's research could be incredibly

helpful at the inquest and trial, and her film was going to be a godsend in getting public attention for change. Despite my serious misgivings about Vanessa's privacy and my family's I told Erna I would go on camera. We planned to film the last three days of January in my home office.

Then, on December 21, I got an early Christmas present from the *Los Angeles Times*. The *Times* had published a series of articles on the drug industry and the FDA that week that exposed regulatory secrecy and failures.[1] One of the articles was on Prepulsid. I sat dumbfounded staring at my screen that morning reading and rereading the detail in David Willman's story, "Drug after Drug, Warnings Ignored."

Before approval in 1993, more than 2 per cent of patients who took Prepulsid in U.S. studies experienced "heart rate and rhythm disorders." One out of fifty.

During the same studies, *eight children aged six and under had died while on Prepulsid.* An FDA report claimed "no clear evidence" implicated Prepulsid, but neither could its role be excluded. Naturally I wondered how often children die during trials for drugs that treat non-life threatening conditions. And I thought children were rarely included in drug trials? Nevertheless, this is the kind of critical safety information that Health Canada should have known about, but were they still keeping it secret to protect Johnson & Johnson's "commercial rights?"

How did Prepulsid get approved in the U.S.? Back in August 1993, the director of the FDA's cardiology division, Dr. Raymond J. Lipicky, cautioned doctors in the *American Journal of Cardiology* that any drug that prolonged QT and had a benefit that was "less than lifesaving . . . any risk of death would likely be considered unacceptable." Yet no one had asked him, or anyone else in the FDA Cardiac Division, to review Prepulsid despite the FDA warning in 1990 that two allergy drugs, Seldane and Hismanal, prolonged the QT interval and posed a lethal risk. Prepulsid was approved by the FDA's Gastrointestinal Division.

In August of 1996 the FDA specifically turned Janssen down for Prepulsid use in children. This was kept secret for competitive commercial reasons. Prepulsid became the drug of choice for infant reflux anyway: the North American Society for Pediatric Gastroenterology and Nutrition promoted Prepulsid as safe and effective for children in their literature, and held a 1998 symposium on the use of Prepulsid in Orlando, Florida. The group had received no strings attached "educational grants" from Janssen. One year later, in August 1997, an FDA director cited three child deaths related to Prepulsid and warned a Janssen official verbally that the FDA might contraindicate its use in infants. This was also kept secret from doctors and patients, and Janssen negotiated another label change ten months later in June 1998. The label read "Causality has not been established."

"And cigarettes do not cause lung cancer," I thought.

There was one more revelation: The *Times* said Prepulsid had been cited as *suspect in 302 deaths*—more than three times the official U.S. number of eighty I'd read so many times.

I couldn't reach Gary Will on the phone but excitedly emailed the article to him. This exposé would have a huge impact at our civil trial.

But a Canadian jury would want to know how Health Canada handled Prepulsid. When I had first started investigating how Vanessa died, regulatory documents I found had been produced by the Health Protection Branch. But some time shortly after that the people in charge of prescription drugs at Health Canada had adopted the name Therapeutic Products Program. The key word "protection" was gone. I called Dr. Michele Brill-Edwards to ask about it.

"From the time the Bureau of Drug Research closed in

1997, our drug reviewers were directed to treat the drug companies as partners, and forced to depend on Big Pharma documentation to determine the safety and effectiveness of their own drugs," she said. "And the companies began to pay millions of dollars in fees to get their drugs reviewed."

My research since revealed that by 2005 more than 60 per cent of the budget for drug reviews was paid by Big Pharma.

"The government of the day also thought it was OK for drug reviewers to meet in closed-door sessions with senior drug company staff, where no minutes were taken," Michele said.

As a former MPP this stopped me cold. Imagine if you saw a judge from your civil trial coming out of a private meeting with the person you were suing for damages. If exposed, that would lead to an immediate mistrial. Well, drug reviewers are a kind of judge. They are supposed to judge if a drug is safe and effective or not, with no undue influence. Hundreds of millions of dollars are often at stake. Company officials should have nothing to say to drug reviewers at private meetings. The very idea implies pressure—or something worse.

Was taking "protection" out of the branch's name just a coincidence? In 1991, the five historic public policy objectives and considerations for drug policy for Canada were: the public health system; consumer protection; relationship to industrial policy; intellectual property; and Canada's multinational relations.[2]

By December 18, 1996, when drug patent legislation was under review, a memorandum to the Cabinet listed the public policy objectives for drug patent policy:

1. Support for the development of the pharmaceutical industry in Canada
2. Ensure patented drugs are available to consumers at non-excessive prices
3. Ensure conformity with Canada's multinational relations

Protection was missing. Public health was missing. Consumer was missing. All replaced with Big Pharma sales priorities.

Here are some examples I've found since showing how Health Canada and our federal government had abandoned safety and embraced their new role as marketing partners of Big Pharma since the mid-nineties.

Senior staff pressured conscientious drug reviewers like Michele Brill-Edwards to approve drugs faster, went over their heads to approve drugs that the reviewers did not find safe, and made their working lives so miserable they had to quit.[3] I can think of two key jobs where you do not want the bosses or politicians to pressure civil servants to hurry up, because getting it right is far more important than doing it quickly. The first is an air traffic controller. The second is a drug reviewer. No one would dream of standing over an air traffic controller at the start of their shift saying, "Get those planes in faster."

Health Canada eliminated others who stood up against unsafe drugs. From 1997 until 2002, four long-term Health Canada scientists wrote to the public service integrity office and every health minister about drugs they saw as unsafe and mad cow disease. Health Canada demoted and eventually fired three of them: Shiv Chopra, Margaret Heydon, and Gerard Lambert. Later in 2004, Chris Bassude, the fourth scientist died prematurely of a suspected heart attack after being demoted.[4]

In May 2003, Health Canada hired an independent "neutral facilitator"[5]—the Public Policy Forum (PPF)—to conduct a stakeholder consultation on "improving Canada's regulatory process." I was to discover that this was pharma-speak for how to get drugs approved faster, a risky practice. I was concerned from the beginning. The board of directors of PPF included the deputy minister of health, Ian C. Green, and Alex Himelfarb, Canada's highest-ranking civil servant. Why were these two on a governance committee for a private organization? Was it not a conflict of interest for them to "hire" a private organization they helped govern to conduct a consultation for the taxpayers? And how could the Public Policy Forum claim to be independent?

I quickly concluded that the advantage of using a third party was that the government could escape accountability. If the opposition or media attacked the outcome of the consultation, the minister could say, "It wasn't us that came with this stuff." But if the media and public were supportive they could take credit. I was invited to participate, and my condition for attending the stakeholder session in an Ottawa hotel was that a number of other drug safety advocates also be invited. They complied. On the first day we knew by 11 a.m. the fix was in. First, no journalists were present. I was bemused because the materials PPF had sent us declared transparency and openness as the second most important principle in the regulatory process. My experience in politics was that when no media are invited the results are going to be "spun" beyond all recognition.[6] Researcher Alan Cassels was present and twice raised the issue of potential conflicts of interest, suggesting those present declare any they might have. That wasn't on. And the moderator, Dr. Jan Elliott, Ph.D., kept responding to our concerns by saying they had no agenda. This was very strange, as the 2002 Throne Speech committed the government to "smart regulation" in part to "speed up the regulatory process for drug approvals." The 2003 federal budget put $190 million on the table to "improve the timeliness" of drug approvals.[7] In fact PPF's own number one objective was listed in the printed materials: "improve timeliness and transparency of regulatory reviews."

So they *had* an agenda.

But their second objective stopped me cold: "Provide greater vigilance around safety issues *once products reach the market* [my italics] including through enhanced post-market surveillance."[8] That was right off Big Pharma's to-do list. After products reach the market! The government was preparing to abandon proving drugs were safe *before* patients took them. This was "smart regulation." Fly now. Pay later.

Big Pharma already had our drug "judges" as partners. But with this proposal they could get their drugs on the market faster, and see if they are safe later. That's risk management. Patients get the risk. They get the management.

The session itself was dominated with another language—bureaucratic double-speak—one I was familiar with as a former MPP. Jan promised to write down what the participants said on big pieces of paper on a tripod, then tape them on the walls around the room, to be collected later and recorded. But she would simply not repeat or write down what we said. It was rather comical, but she managed to keep a straight face.

One of the safety advocates said faster approvals compromise safety. She wrote down "timeliness" on the big piece of paper on the tripod. Someone said secrecy was a cause of repeated adverse reactions from new drugs. She wrote down "proprietary contents" underneath "timeliness." I said that "corrupt practices" in the industry were leading to unsafe drugs being approved. She wrote down "management practices." And so it went.[9]

Later, PPF consulted with other "stakeholders" on other days, including the drug industry, and "disease-awareness" groups (many of them funded in part by the industry). The PPF final report declared the number one critical direction: "Consider the regulatory system for therapeutic products to be a national resource, and develop and invest in it accordingly."[10] The word "safety" didn't even appear in their top three priorities. Pushing safety down the list of priorities was evident in every significant undertaking I saw at Health Canada in those years.

We attended the Christmas Eve service at midnight at St. Jude's in Oakville. As I sat in the crowded candlelit church beside Hart, Gloria, and Madeline, I tried very hard to reconcile my faith with Vanessa's death. Why did this happen? Could it be part of God's plan? I always believed God gave mankind stewardship of this world—and our independence. People make choices every day between right and wrong. Occasionally we must choose between self interest—profit, higher share value or a year-end bonus—and doing what is right. Sometimes people make the wrong choices. And these choices can play out on the innocent. It wasn't God's fault.

That was all I could come up with. For the time being, it would have to do.

But I prayed the inquest and coming trial would expose exactly who had made the wrong choices.

We gathered with our extended families over the holiday, talking, eating, exchanging gifts, even laughing. But the empty space in our family was there, and I wondered if I would ever see my family experience joy again. Over the holiday I resolved to do my utmost to try to protect them from revisiting our tragedy day to day. I'd keep it to myself, I figured. But Erna's film crew arriving at the house at the end of January wasn't going to help.

CBC producer Rene Pellerin had sent me a video copy of *Marketplace*, originally broadcast in November 1999, featuring her investigation of a thirty-seven-year-old mother of three who died in Halifax on May 4, 1998, after taking Prepulsid with a contraindicated drug—the antibiotic erythromycin. The Health Canada Chief of Post-market Surveillance, Chris Turner, had been interviewed for *Marketplace*: "As long as the patient is making an informed decision," he said, "then we feel the manufacturer has taken adequate action." It saddened me to hear this. Health Canada decision-makers knew very well patients and doctors were *not* making informed decisions with Prepulsid in November 1998, a year before this program was aired. I had their meeting minutes that proved that most doctors didn't even know if Prepulsid was safe.

I was very curious about Anna Kovacs' claim about drugs: "The patients think it was the drug that helped them. They believe it, so the doctors believe it." How could patients feel better if a drug had no real effect?

It's called placebo.

I spent many evenings researching placebo. A front-page story *The New York Times Magazine* had published a year before, entitled "The Placebo Prescription," asked this question: Since placebos work, why aren't we prescribing them?

A placebo is nothing. A dummy pill. A ruse. Taken orally it is usually a sugar pill, or water in a capsule. Yet time and time again in drug trials where the patients don't know what they are taking, the number of patients who report relief from their symptoms from placebos is the same as the number of patients on the real drug.

Placebos are reported to work on average 33 per cent of the time. A third of patients taking sugar pills actually believe the pills are addressing their symptoms. The power of suggestion creates a kind of counterfeit value for many patients, and keeps them coming back for more.

In 2003 a leading expert on prescription drugs made an astonishing statement at a scientific meeting in London, England. Dr. Allen Roses, vice-president of genetics for GlaxoSmithKline (GSK), the world's second-largest drug company reported, "The vast majority of drugs—more than 90 percent—only work in 30 or 50 percent of people." GSK marketed the blockbusters Advair, Avandia, Paxil, Zophran, Wellbutrin, and Augmentin.

To read Dr. Roses' frank admission was amazing. Executives of the major drug companies are normally extremely careful with what they say about their drugs, because any offhand comment might cause the company stock to drop, end up as evidence in a lawsuit against the company, or hurt sales. But this executive was stating publicly that their products were useless for more than a third of their customers. They'd be better off with little capsules full of water. So why did they keep taking them? Because, I learned, the action of getting a prescription from a trusted doctor and swallowing the drug was powerful enough to make them feel better. From a blockbuster viewpoint, the placebo effect makes winners out of losers.

Other than the so-called natural health products, what other products in the world have such a dismal success rate? Imagine if appliances only worked properly two-thirds of the time. What if you could only eat two-thirds of the food you bought? The difference is that because of the placebo effect, it's very hard to tell when prescription drugs *aren't* working. Anna Kovacs also said, "Who's to tell them otherwise?" The placebo effect doesn't just fool patients. It fools doctors.

Prescription drugs sales hit the $600 billion mark world-wide in 2006. Dr. Roses was saying indirectly that perhaps $200 billion a year spent worldwide on prescription drugs is really wasted. And since all drugs cause adverse reactions, millions of patients are put at risk daily for no good reason.

Why don't we prescribe placebos? The answer is simple: effectively, we are. Only they have brand names.

Chapter 14

Physician, Heal Thyself

*"There is no greater calamity greater than lavish desires.
There is no greater guilt than discontentment.
And there is no greater disaster than greed."*
—Lao-tzu (604 BC–531 BC)

"There is gold for you. Sell me your good report."
—William Shakespeare, *Cymbeline*

January 2, 2001

I STARTED THE SECOND DAY of the new year sitting in my
housecoat at 8 a.m. reading the *Globe and Mail*. Journalist
Krista Foss explained how drug companies spent an estimated
one billion dollars a year marketing to our doctors in Canada.[1]
The marketing included "drug samples to salsa lessons, wine
tastings to expensive free trips to exotic climes ..." In exchange
for some of their time for "continuing medical education"
(CME) Bayer Canada had taken a bunch of doctors to a country
club for golf and a brewery tour and dinner. Janssen-Ortho and

Schering-Plough paid for a weekend getaway for a group of doctors—three days at a four-star ski resort in the Laurentians—if they attended some workshops there. This, I read, is "continuing medical education."

Doctors could even get cash payments for ghostwriting research papers, or lending their name to papers written by someone else—just the kind of thing that would have gotten them kicked out of medical school!

They could get between one and two thousand dollars simply for attending "advisory board" meetings or "focus groups." Larger fees were available for "thought leaders" who spoke at CMA events. Twenty thousand dollars' worth of stuff on average was being given to, or spent per doctor yearly by the most profitable companies in the world.

Corporations don't give money away out of kindness.

IS YOUR DOCTOR CHEATING ON YOU?

You may think the relationship with your doctor is almost sacred. You trust him or her totally. However, it is likely that there is a member of your healthcare team you will never see who has huge influence over the care you receive: Big Pharma. Big Pharma executives will tell you with a straight face that their primary concern is for safety. But their most important marketing strategy is to create a profitable relationship with the person who makes the buying decision: your doctor. Unfortunately these relationships are primarily about sales, not science.

They start by never calling anything what it is. Any term that might even sound like sales or marketing is transformed into a pharma-speak euphemism outside their sales office. For example, continuing medical education is usually a disguised sales seminar, with free booze and gourmet food, often in a posh location. But they also have their own in-house language that reveals the true nature of their business. I'll translate each pharma-speak term the first time I use it.

"Detail reps" is pharma-speak for sales reps or drug reps. Sales is their job. Every doctor has a copy of the *CPS* in his office—the *Compendium of Pharmaceuticals and Specialties*—which contains the official prescribing information, or label, for most drugs. There is no shortage of detail available in drug labels, which can exceed thirty pages.[2] But those labels contain a lot of details the drug companies don't want your doctor to discover—like the numbers of ADRs reported during clinical trials, awful side effects, or that almost as many patients on placebos reported benefits as those on the drug. Big Pharma prefers to have their cheerful sales reps out there singing the praises of their drugs—over a catered lunch they brought along for the doctor and his staff.

Unfortunately our doctors' reliance on these marketing relationships divides their loyalty, and influences everything they hear about prescription drugs—and don't hear. I spent a great deal of time reading about how our doctors are influenced by the pharmaceutical companies. It was discouraging.

First, most doctors rely on Big Pharma drug reps for most of their information on new drugs. The drug reps grab any time they might get—even a few minutes between patient appointments. They also visit our medical schools, hospitals, and doctors' offices to pitch their drugs using sales techniques with pharma-speak names like "mental shortcuts"—a sales process designed to bypass the doctor's critical thought.[3]

Detail reps' favourite doctors are called "wolves"—those that are more influenced by gifts and are primarily concerned with making money.[4] It's harder to sell to "sheep"—who are more conformist doctors, but are influenced by expert testimonials. "Bunnies" are progressive doctors who might respond to dramatic emotional messages about suffering, or the drug's benefits. Then there are the doctors they call "dodos"—burned-out docs trying to survive.

Second, Alan Cassels was so right: Big Pharma dominates every other source doctors rely on for information about prescription drugs—funding most research and financing experts they call "thought leaders." Even the *CPS* has full-page colour drug ads. And I discovered that if the drug companies don't pay to put a drug in the *CPS*, it's not there. That's why the drugs that have been taken off the market for harming patients like Prepulsid tend to disappear as if they never existed. That's influence.

In the months after Vanessa's death I connected with a number of former drug reps. Most of them wouldn't reveal anything about their former jobs. One who did was Callie Hughes, who lobbied me when I was MPP in the late nineties. Like many other former detail reps, after a time she found drug detailing to be highly unethical and left the industry. Her frank admissions held me spellbound.

She told me how their marketing chief used to fire up the troops before they headed out to their territories. They zeroed in on the high-scrip docs: "This is a good drug. Ask them why they aren't writing scrips for it. Get a commitment from them to write a specific number of scrips per month!" And that's what she and her colleagues did. But in Callie's case it wasn't just the doctors. The generic companies also focus on high-volume pharmacists, and her company bought the pharmacist's sales information from data companies. So Callie could actually monitor how many scrips for each drug came out of each pharmacy. Her job was getting the pharmacists to switch the patients to their version of the drug. Callie described the method:

"I kept electronic appliances in the back of my car—a TV, a VCR, a fax machine. I would say to the pharmacist 'Tell me what you want in order to switch your patients to our drug. I'll go get it from my car right now.'"

I asked her if those methods worked.

"You're darn right they worked. I did it many times. And other detail reps were doing the same thing with the doctors."

Researcher Alan Cassels tells the story of Mike Oldani, Ph.D., a former drug sales rep, now an anthropologist and professor at the University of Wisconsin at Whitewater. Like most detail reps. Mike kept electronic files on each of the physicians in his sales area including not only what drugs each doctor prescribed, but his own notes on their likes and dislikes, their spouses' and children's birthdays, and their favourite wines. He knew what motivated his doctors. This is a common practice in the industry, openly admitted to by many detail reps. To help curry favour many also track personal details of people working in doctor's offices.[5]

"The importance of developing loyalty through gifting cannot be overstated," writes Mike Oldani.[6] "The essence of pharmaceutical gifting is 'bribes that aren't considered bribes.'"[7]

Former Eli Lilly detail rep Shahram Ahari describes a detail rep's job as changing the prescribing habits of physicians. "It's my job to figure out what a physician's price is. For some it's dinner at the finest restaurants, for others it's enough convincing data to let them prescribe confidently and for others it's my attention and friendship . . . but at the most basic level, everything is for sale and everything is an exchange."[8]

Drug reps are well paid. The average annual salary for a drug rep by 2004 was $64,200 with a car and benefits, plus $19,300 in bonuses.[9] The bottom line: the more their doctors prescribe their pills, the more they earn. I've sold a lot of different products and services over a twenty-five-year business career: cars, boats, telephone systems, and more. No matter what anyone says, people whose career and pay depend on sales do not raise the weaknesses of their products. Everyone knows car salesmen are paid on commission. They tell you the good stuff about their product. But they do not normally raise engineering faults or recalls. Drug reps are no different.

They are more like cheerleaders who are given limited information—all the good stuff—and sent out to increase sales. They are not bad people. Many of them really believe what they are saying.[10] Others do what they have to do.

One evening I called Alan Cassels at his home in Victoria to ask about this. He laughed a little. "Drug reps are trained to 'spin-doctor' the drawbacks of their drugs in a positive way. For example, for a drug that can make patients drowsy and unable to drive safely the drug rep might say 'It helps patients sleep.' For a drug that causes nausea, they might say 'It helps patients lose weight.'"

Some people may think, "That's just business. All businesses do that. Doctors are wise enough to know when they're hearing biased information, and not getting the full safety story." But the evidence shows they aren't.

Former detail reps have gone on record about how the truth is tortured when drug reps talk to our doctors, and how the safety stuff is left out. Sometimes they give them outright false information, and the doctors believe it. An article from the *Journal of the American Medical Association* in April 1995, entitled "The accuracy of drug information from pharmaceutical representatives,"[11] reported that researchers recorded 106 statements made by drug reps about their drugs at presentations to resident doctors at a university teaching hospital. Even though they were being recorded, more than 10 per cent of the statements the reps made were inaccurate—all favourable to the drug. Later, only 26 per cent of the doctors recalled any false statement. But 37 per cent said drug rep information influenced the way they prescribe drugs! Having been in sales for many years, I naturally wondered how accurate the detail reps' claims would be when they were *not* being recorded.

In 1998, researcher Dr. Joel Lexchin found strong links between more doctor–drug rep contact, and increased inappropriate prescribing. Doctors who saw drug reps more often favoured a "commercial" view of drugs rather than the view in the scientific literature, and prescribed more expensive drugs when cheaper and equally effective drugs were available. That could certainly influence the therapy of vulnerable elderly people.

Indeed, according to a report in the *Journal of the American Medical Association*, doctors that had accepted financial support from a drug company were ten times more likely to request their drug be added to the hospital formulary.[12] *Ten times.*

Does drug "detailing" work? In 1997 Warner-Lambert marketed their "me too" drug that lowers cholesterol, Lipitor, to outsell the leading cholesterol-lowering drug, Zocor. A small army of Warner detail reps went out and visited 81,000 doctors "every month for several months,"[13] pitching its strength and newness, and succeeded in pushing Lipitor over the top to number one.

Detailing works, big-time.

But the biggest safety problem is off-label promotion. In August 2004, Warner-Lambert (now owned by Pfizer) pleaded guilty to fraudulent promotion of its epilepsy drug Neurontin (gabapentin) and paid a fine of $430 million to "resolve" criminal and civil charges against its Parke-Davis Division (no one went to jail). They had promoted Neurontin for a dozen uses for which it was never approved, including some that had been proven to be ineffective.[14] They made illegal kickbacks to thousands of doctors.[15] They also paid doctors to come on lavish trips to places like Puerto Rico and Hawaii, and even paid $350 *for allowing the sales rep to visit them.* One doctor received almost $308,000 to tout Neurontin at conferences. Here is a quote from Parke-Davis executive John Ford taken from a recorded meeting of his marketing managers in April 1996: "Dinner programs, CME [continuing medical education], consultantships—all work great, but don't forget the one-on-one. That's where we need to be, holding their hand and whispering in their ear, Neurontin for pain, Neurontin for monotherapy, Neurontin for bipolar, Neurontin for everything...I don't want to see a single patient coming off Neurontin before they've been up to at least 4800 milligrams a day...I don't want to hear that safety crap either—every one of you should take one just to see there is nothing. It's great drug."[16]

By 2003 Neurontin was almost triple blockbuster with $2.7 billion in sales. Like Prepulsid, a large portion of its sales were off-label.[17] Unfortunately, over 258 suicides of patients on Neurontin were individually reported to the FDA Medwatch by March 2005. Over 2,300 families are now taking legal steps against Pfizer because they blame Neurontin for a suicide or suicide attempt of a loved one.[18]

Sometimes I picture a vulnerable Canadian senior like my mother heading into her doctor's office, trusting totally he would recommend the best therapy for her. She would carefully outline her symptoms while he took her blood pressure. What if this vulnerable lady was truly better off without a drug? How would she stand a chance against all the Big Pharma enticements?

How did so many doctors get from "Do no Harm" to "Don't look a gift-horse in the mouth"? In the ensuing weeks I learned the drug companies get to our doctors long before they swear to "do no harm."

Chapter 15

Get 'em While
They're Young

"Gratitude is merely the secret hope of further favors."
—Francois de La Rochefoucauld

*In October 2003, a fifteen-year-old girl was killed by a pre-
scription drug. Tiffany Whitter, of Wickler, Manitoba, loved to
sing, and once won a singing competition singing Sarah
McLachlan's "Angel." She was known for her radiant smile and
how she befriended everybody. Manitoba's chief medical exam-
iner confirmed in May 2004 that she had died of cardiac arrest—a preventable death—caused by Duragesic, a pain-relief
patch she never should have been prescribed.*

    *Like Prepulsid, Duragesic is a Janssen-Ortho/Johnson &
Johnson blockbuster. Duragesic was not recommended for children under eighteen or anyone not already tolerating a narcotic-
based pain reliever like Tylenol 3.*

    *Health Canada had received voluntary reports of over 31
deaths related to Duragesic as far back as 1993, so the true number could be higher. I called Tiffany's father and we chatted. The*

Whitters had no warning about Duragesic from their doctor or pharmacist.

Three years after Vanessa died and nothing had changed.[1]

JANUARY WAS BUSY FOR ME with client work and adjudicating hearings for the Alcohol and Gaming Commission. Some hearings were "agreed," and settled by 11:30 a.m., and others went until late afternoon, or into another day. I used any spare time to prepare for the inquest and coming trial. Erna Buffie was planning to bring her film crew into my home office on January 25th to interview me. Some time in January I realized that would be a mistake. Bringing my battle into the privacy of our home was not a good idea. Madeline was at Queen's in Kingston, but this might reopen old wounds for Gloria and Hart. I called Erna the day before and we moved the filming to another location.

But we did film a few minutes behind our house in the snowy ravine—I was throwing snowballs in the air for our golden retriever Romulus to catch in his mouth, a game he enjoyed. It felt surreal to me that Vanessa's favourite pet was here playing with me, and she wasn't. She loved him so much. A Christmas Eve years before flooded my memory—a joyous time. I had been there in the ravine dressed in a Santa Claus costume Gloria had made, carrying a big red sack. I climbed the hill behind the house to wave in the moonlight over the back fence to Madeline, Vanessa, and Hart inside. The children's excitement as they ran off to bed was contagious. Heading back down I slipped in the snow, down onto one knee, and paused to remove some burrs caught in my white beard. A white rabbit, perfectly camouflaged in the snow, sat motionless staring at me. Life was so beautiful—like a dream to me. This was my new reality—trying to understand and expose the faults of this complex regulatory system. I so wanted my old life back.

The inquest was less than two months away. Gary had said that our civil case would be primarily based on the inadequate Canadian Prepulsid warnings, particularly the fact that Canadians did not get the same black box warning in 1998 that Americans did. But I feared that Vanessa's reputation would come under attack at the inquest.

We had submitted what I felt was irrefutable evidence to the coroner, like the *Los Angeles Times* exposé. I wanted to tell the jury how eight children had died during clinical trials for Prepulsid, and that doctors ignore the warnings. We had also submitted copies of the minutes of the Health Canada Pharmacovigilance meeting from November 1998 which discussed how inadequate the warnings were.

So in mid-February I was somewhat cheered as Gary Will and I headed into a pre-inquest conference at the courthouse to meet with Brian O'Marra, the Crown attorney who would assist the coroner at the inquest, and the lawyers for two of the other parties that had also been given "standing" to participate in the inquest.

But I felt a little panicked when Brian O'Marra told us that the coroner had deemed some of our key evidence inadmissible.

"A great deal of evidence had been submitted from the various parties," he said. "A lot of it goes beyond what the jury will need to determine a cause of death and make their recommendations. An inquest can't go on for months. The jury will read and hear evidence only on the relevant facts in this death."

This was a disaster.

How could the jury make recommendations to prevent similar deaths if they didn't know how the actions of the various parties kept this dangerous drug on the market with ineffective warnings? I thought the coroner had lost his mind. Anyone could read that information and see it was highly relevant. What was going on?

I hoped Mr. O'Marra would try to change the coroner's mind, and pleaded with him: "We've spent months gathering information on safety warnings that is highly relevant to potential jury recommendations, and to why Vanessa died."

"An inquest is limited by law to deal with specific questions, issues and recommendations," he explained to me firmly. "It is not and cannot be a wide-ranging judicial inquiry or Royal Commission. Nor is it a process for redress of wrongs or allegations. I'm sure all relevant information can be introduced."

I doubted it. Were we supposed to call up FDA experts quoted in the *Times* and ask them politely to fly up to Hamilton, Ontario, in March to act as witnesses? Even if they agreed, who would pay for that? And I highly doubted anyone from Health Canada—who we were suing—would provide testimony helpful to me and Vanessa.

Gary maintained his composure as he discussed administrative details of the inquest with Mr. O'Marra and the other lawyers, but could see I was distressed. Then we said our goodbyes. In the parking lot we stood beside Gary's car in the cold February wind, as he explained to me what had just happened.

"The role of the Crown in an inquest is not like in a criminal trial. He is not an advocate for any party or interest. He is Counsel to the coroner. The coroner is aware of the stakes for the parties in this case. He knows the parties view the inquest as a warmup for a coming civil trial. This is high-profile. That's why he's going to be scrupulously fair in making sure the process does not exceed its legal limits. Finding fault is not this jury's duty. But I think the coroner wants to get good recommendations." He gave me a half-smile. Confident though. "There are other ways to get our evidence in front of the jury."

"How?" I asked.

"Through witnesses."

Nothing seemed to faze Gary. Still, I was distraught as I drove home. I suspected the coroner would stop Gary when he tried to bring in evidence he'd *already* deemed irrelevant.

And if the coroner didn't think that the *Times* article and Health Canada meeting minutes were relevant, what *else* might he decide was not relevant? After months of incremental progress, for the first time I felt I might fail. I could lose. They might get away with it. All of them.

I'd been leading my double life now since the summer. Since Christmas I'd stopped talking at home about every new un-savoury practice I'd uncovered about the drug industry, or change in the status of our case, expecting my family to get excited about it. That was a good thing, because at this point I'd have to tell them we were in trouble heading into the inquest. I was afraid we'd be unable to convince the jury that Prepulsid killed Vanessa.

But as a husband and father I was unable to ignore another nagging fear that haunted me—a fear that because the world is a dangerous place, a loved one can die with no warning. No parent is exempt from this reality.

One evening, late, Madeline called from Queen's with a terrible cold. My knee-jerk reaction was to wonder "what if?" and conjure up the worst-case scenario. I had to make sure she did not contract meningitis overnight. I had no reason to think she would. In fact, I knew I was overreacting—being irrational. Gloria knew exactly where my head—and heart—was, and didn't try to dissuade me. At 5 a.m. I drove three and a half hours to Kingston. Madeline came down to open the student residence door in her housecoat with a stuffy nose. It was just a cold. Non-emergency over. I told Madeline I'd drive as far as Vancouver if she needed me. We chatted for a while, hugged, and I headed back home—wondering if fear would be my default position for any unexpected health symptom the rest of my life.

That evening I logged onto www.nofreelunch.org. The site was created by Dr. Bob Goodman and like-minded colleagues at Columbia University Medical Centre in New York, because they were fed up with the gifts pharmaceutical companies were giving medical students and doctors. The personal stories gave me tremendous insight into why our doctors feel it's acceptable to accept the many corporate gifts from the pharmaceutical companies.

Most medical schools, supposed to be dedicated to objective science, allow drug company reps to freely walk their hallways, from their first week of classes.[2] Their strategy is to get to the students before they've developed their lifelong prescribing habits, which are hard to break later.[3] They want them to equate health with drugs, and begin to trust and rely on drug reps for their drug information. They start by buying them pizza lunches, tickets to events, and sometimes their first leather medical bag on graduation day. This creates layers of problems later that undermine our health.

First, drugs as therapy are over-represented in medical schools. Drugs are all they hear about over free lunches—not other therapies. And drug reps don't balance their hype by recounting the many drug disasters, from thalidomide to fen-phen[4] to Prepulsid.

Second, medical students kick off their careers as scientists doing something very unscientific and naive—trusting highly biased sources for information crucial to our health. A scientist is always supposed to rely on the best available *objective* information.

Third, they pick up muddled ethical thinking from their teachers and administrators, developing a sense of entitlement— the belief that someone, somewhere, owes them. If you are entitled, gifts are not a bribe. Those who provide your entitlement will always get the facetime, won't they? But that means that critical, balanced safety information may never get on the schedule.

Fourth, by accepting a gift, even a free lunch, they are accepting a debt of gratitude. One of the most powerful social rules in our society is to return favours to those who are nice to us.[5] It's human nature. And it is not necessarily limited to the size of the gift. Either consciously or subconsciously, doctors who accept gifts are joining a network of obligation.[6] And what is the only way a doctor can ever pay back that debt to a drug rep? Try their new drugs—experiment—on you.

Fifth, most medical students and doctors don't believe the gifts change what they prescribe for their patients. A major study in the *Journal of the American Medical Association* in January 2000 analyzed twenty-nine published articles since 1994. It concluded that the free trips and Big Pharma presentations were associated with "nonrational prescribing" of the sponsor's medications—increased prescriptions of their drugs.[7] Most medical residents and doctors denied that gifts could influence their behaviour.

The doctors think they are immune from debts of gratitude. So, *they are being influenced but don't know it.* They will look their colleagues right in the eye and say the gifts and free trips and money are irrelevant. That is a drug rep's dream.

About 80 to 95 per cent of doctors see Big Pharma salespeople regularly,[8] normally up to four times a month. There are about 100,000 full-time sales reps in North America employed by the pharmaceutical companies[9] and about 682,000 practicing physicians.[10] That's about one drug rep for every seven practicing doctors. But drug reps focus on the 20 per cent that are high-scrip docs, so the effective ratio is far lower—about one sales rep for every 1.5 high-scrip doctors. The sales reps give medical residents an average of six gifts a year. Smaller gifts can be fountain pens, paper pads, day timers, textbooks, or brief-cases. Even the smaller gifts can influence your care—for example, patient handouts or education posters that omit important safety information.

This is so strange, in my view. After all, who trusts door-to-door salespeople? Yet according to the *New England Journal of Medicine*, Big Pharma spends $15 billion to $20 billion a year sending out door-to-door sales reps to influence our doctors—between $8,000 to $15,000 per doctor.[11] But the pens and pads and briefcases only represent the thin edge of the wedge. In time free knick-knacks can morph into catered lunches, expensive dinners, golf games, admissions to hockey games or other high-end events, travel expenses, and payments to attend pharma-sponsored events.

The weird thing is, drug reps are not hired for their profound understanding of pharmacology (how drugs work in the body). Prized or requisite skills—as outlined in a Merck career brochure—are "sales and persuasion skills, communication, leadership, planning and organization, self-motivation and initiative."[12] Eli Lilly calls for reps with a "return on investment mentality."[13]

Has your doctor ever handed you a free sample of an over-the-counter or prescription drug? Well, the few packets of drugs your doctor has given you and others add up $8 billion a year on free samples.[14] No industry gives away that much product to be nice. They expect the patients that try those drugs to come back and ask for more. Boosted by the powerful placebo effect, the patients usually feel better, so free samples start millions of patients taking the latest blockbuster drugs. But most of the free samples are the most expensive drugs, and some patients can't keep paying for them. And once started on a drug it may be hard to change later. Also, the free sample box contains the latest, not the most effective drugs, and may not be exactly what is required.

So some poor soul gets a few free packets. If he can't afford to buy the stuff long-term, or it's not the best drug for him, how is he better off?

In reality, I think it's the doctors who are being manipulated with free samples. They are the ones with the biggest debts of gratitude—accepting billions in free samples to please their patients. The only way they can "pay" the drug reps back? By writing out prescriptions that will put their drugs into our bloodstreams and organs.

Medical journals have expressed concern about this: the professional relationship is one between two unequal parties, where the party with more power has the responsibility for the well-being of the other.[15] Your doctor's sworn loyalty is to act in your best interest and protect you from harm. That should mean using the best available objective evidence to decide what is best for you, period.

There is no taking gifts or money on the side for a judge. There is no third-party "wink wink, here's some free stuff for your family" for professional umpires or referees. There is no "Hey professor, let me take you to Cannes where I'll tell you why I deserve an 'A' this term." Any of these professionals could lose their job for taking gifts. For a chuckle, think about this: Ironically, even drug reps are not allowed to accept any gifts![16] Yet doctors are openly enticed.

But the Big Pharma companies are not satisfied with directly influencing our doctors. Doctors are taught in medical school to trust three main sources of information: continuing medical education, medical journals, and their peers. Big Pharma has carefully invested their wealth to undermine the objectivity of all three. Big Pharma pays for about three-quarters of all continuing medical education (CME) events. They even fund 63.8 per cent of the CME in medical schools.[17] No drug rep ever speaks at a sponsored CME event. They hire credible speakers—

"thought leaders"—other doctors or researchers they are paying to come in and lecture our doctors.

Drug-sponsored CME has one key purpose: to get their favourite "thought leaders" in front of a group of well-fed, relaxed and much-indebted docs. The best way is by holding some CME sessions in some pretty exotic places.[18] AstraZeneca seems to have been caught breaking the rules the most, and was put on probation and fined by its own industry association, Rx&D, in 2005 for an "unprecedented" number of violations of the group's code of ethical conduct. In 2003 they'd taken a bunch of doctors to the Ritz Carlton in Jamaica, and then another lucky group to Cannes, France. AstraZeneca VP Sheila Frame was quoted in the *Globe and Mail* referring to the infractions as mostly technicalities: "The infractions themselves are not something we're embarrassed about. There is nothing unethical in the infractions."

This is an issue fundamental to our health and safety. To a drug company, every disease or condition is a way to sell a drug. They aren't paying hundreds of millions of dollars to spend time with doctors so they'll persuade patients to exercise, quit smoking without drugs, or how they can lower cholesterol with diet changes. They aren't inviting chiropractors to come in and talk to doctors about how drug-free care and massage can reduce pain. They aren't financing CME seminars on how one can beat depression with talk therapy and whole range of safer activities that millions of people have found helpful like gardening, music therapy, grief counselling, or a daily dose of sunshine.

And they aren't there to caution our doctors about adverse drug reactions.

If anyone asks a question about adverse reactions at a pharma-sponsored CME event the "thought leader" will often craft the messaging by saying the effects are small, or only affect a subset of patients, and that they resolve over time. They might say something like "and oh, by the way, causes liver failure in a small number of patients."[19] Next slide please.

They leave an awful lot out. The problem is that half the truth is a whole lie.

On April 27, 2006 Rx&D Chair Paul Lucas, also Canadian president for GlaxoSmithKline, spoke at the Mississauga Board of Trade on the proposed National Pharmaceutical Strategy—which would establish national standards and prices for drugs—and Ontario's Bill 102: "We believe the physician relationship with the patient is critical to achieving positive health outcomes." "We need to ensure that Bill 102 protects the integrity of the patient/physician relationship."

This from an industry that spends billions of dollars every year to successfully undermine that very thing.

SECTION FOUR

Unholy Alliances

Chapter 16

Ganging Up on Vanessa

"A political system dependent on charity from corporations managed by rich men isolated from the masses in chauffeur-driven limousines and private jets, with $100 million retirement packages is not a true democracy. It is a kleptocracy." —Peter Rost, M.D., former vp of Pfizer, from "The New Robber Barons," keynote address, 2006 U.S. Prescription Access Litigation dinner

I WAS VERY BUSY the rest of February and the first half of March with client work, and AGCO hearings took me as far away as Ottawa. On March 12th I attended the funeral of Ontario Cabinet Minister Al Palladini. Sadly, Al had died of a heart attack at age fifty-seven. Despite partisan politics, his presence and unforgettable smile would be missed by everyone at Queen's Park, along with everyone who knew him. The church filled with mourners was a stark reminder to me of how fragile life can be, and how I had to make every day count on my own journey.

Day One
Monday, March 19, 2001

Despite everything I had accomplished and learned in the last year—from my first phone call to Health Canada the day after Vanessa died—I was facing the unknown that cloudy March morning as my van joined a river of trucks heading west on the QEW towards Niagara Falls and Fort Erie. I exited onto the 403 and then onto Main Street West into Hamilton—where exactly one year earlier Vanessa had died.

This was the day the province of Ontario would officially begin to find out why. This is what I had wanted, worked for, and needed to obtain some kind of justice for Vanessa.

But the failure of institutions was the reason I was there. Driving past the old converted houses and fast food restaurants on Main Street towards the John Sopinka Courthouse, I wondered if this institution—the Ontario Coroner's office—would fail Vanessa as well. Time seemed to have forgotten downtown Hamilton with its many old four-storey office buildings, and people smoking cigarettes everywhere. You couldn't drive very far without seeing a Tim Hortons coffee shop.

Something else had me deeply worried. Hamilton is a regional health centre, home to McMaster University Medical Centre and medical school, and three other hospitals. Despite being the home of Stelco Steel, health care is Hamilton's number one employer. More people in Hamilton work as doctors, nurses, technicians, maintenance staff, and administrators than in any other area of endeavour. And they all had families and friends. Could a jury composed of Hamilton residents be truly unbiased in deciding if a prescription drug given in error caused Vanessa's death?

The John Sopinka Courthouse is the former Hamilton Post Office building, beautifully renovated in 1999 to accommodate busy criminal, civil, and small claims courts.

I arrived before the building opened at 8:30 a.m., and stood on the front steps with a handful of others who were smoking and drinking coffee from cardboard cups, waiting for the doors to open. Some of the young men had long hair tied back neatly and suits on. Others who hadn't bothered to dress up were in denim and leather jackets. The strain showing on the faces revealed those who might be facing charges.

Lawyers had their own entrance, but when the doors opened I had to line up with the accused, their families, and witnesses to dump out my pockets and pass through a metal detector like airport security. The security guards searched my briefcase and gave me a once-over with a hand-held metal detector as I raised my arms. The lobby was crowded and noisy. A sign over the door said: "All persons entering this court house will be subject to search. All weapons will be confiscated."

It was surreal to be there. I wished the last year had been a long very detailed nightmare that I could now wake up from—like I'd been in a coma. The sixth floor had a spacious open lobby with windows that went from the floor to the ten-foot-high ceiling, providing a superb view of upper Hamilton. Three rows of modern stainless steel chairs were lined back-to-back on a spotless granite floor. I walked the few steps to the door of Courtroom 600, took a deep breath and gently pulled open one of the silent wooden doors to see where fate had brought me. My home for the next few weeks.

It was a brightly lit room, like a large chapel, with high ceilings. From the back there were seven rows of beechwood benches divided by two aisles. The walls were also paneled with beechwood, and grey carpet deadened the sound of footfalls or moving chairs. In front were six tables for counsel in two rows—three on each side, with three chairs facing the front behind each, and slender black microphone stands sticking up from the table tops. In the centre aisle at the front was a lectern with its own microphone. Every word would be recorded.

At the front, facing towards the back was the judge's bench, about five feet high, with a lower bench in front with three chairs. Above the judge's chair on the wall was a hand painted plaque depicting the scales of justice and the emblem of Ontario. Underneath it said "Justicia."

I felt I was playing a part in a play, and I didn't know how it would end. The courtroom was hushed in comparison to the lobby, as the lawyers for the various parties strolled in, rolling their extra-wide briefcases behind them and chatting as they unloaded their heavy briefing books onto the desks. Because we had standing, Gary Will and I were seated at the front on the left-hand side. Gary's articling student, Vanessa Tanner, sat between us—her name another coincidence.

Across the aisle to our right were Brian O'Marra and David Carruthers who represented the Crown, and to their right the empty jury box with five chairs, with a private door in the wall behind.

Gary was shaking hands and chatting with the lawyers who represented the doctors, sitting at the table behind us. The Johnson & Johnson lawyers sat at the table behind Mr. O'Marra on the right, and two Health Canada representatives were at the table behind them. All the parties had standing, and would be able to ask questions of witnesses, and introduce their own witnesses, including us. Detective Constable Kevin Britton from Halton Regional Police Services sat on the right side at the front.

I never felt less control over anything in my life, like I was outside the room, looking in. Like no one could see me. I'd asked for this. I wanted it. Yet I wished I could turn back the clock. I was just a small part of this process that was supposed to tell the world what—or who—killed my little girl. I had done my homework. I didn't fear the truth. I never wanted anything more in my life than this truth to come out. But we were facing very powerful organizations that had their own versions of the truth. I understood the opposition lawyers had a job to do, but I knew Vanessa's reputation was going to be expendable. It's amazing what people can say about you when you're not there to defend yourself. And some of our most important evidence had been deemed irrelevant.

Two public relations professionals were busily identifying themselves to the media people at the back of the courtroom, obviously working for the other side. I found out later that one was from the U.S. and remembered what Gary had said: "We're the first out of the chute for Prepulsid." By now hundreds of Prepulsid actions had been launched in the U.S. and three class actions in Canada. Every lawyer involved would want to know the outcome here.

I tried to rise above it all. I breathed deeply to try to slow my heart. That didn't work. I took off my coat and sat in the front row beside Gary Will and his assistant Vanessa Tanner, and prayed. I asked for help—for Vanessa's sake. If anything displeases God the most, I think it must be when someone allows children to be hurt.

I began to feel an incredibly reassuring presence around me. This never happened to me before and hasn't happened since. I knew that Gary and I and Vanessa Tanner were not alone. I had no doubt. My heart slowed. My breathing evened. I felt I could deal with whatever happened. I took out a thick eight-by-eleven notepad and pen and prepared to take notes. It was about to start.

Everyone stood when the coroner, Dr. David Eden, entered, just like a trial. He controlled and directed everything that happened for the next sixteen days as a judge would have. Erna Buffie was in the spectator benches behind us with others from the media, having been refused the right to film any part of the proceedings. The first order the coroner gave that morning was that no cameras or media interviews would be allowed in or around the building.

Coroner's juries in Ontario are composed of five people. Ours was three women and two men. I was glad. Since more women advocate for drug safety, and more women are care-givers, I felt they'd be more sympathetic to our case. They all looked to be very decent people, and seemed attentive. A good start, I thought. With five, if they were split on any issue, a majority of three would determine the outcome.

In an inquest, the coroner's counsel, the coroner, and even jury members can ask questions. The day passed quickly with evidence of what happened the day Vanessa collapsed. Mr. O'Marra provided a summary of the facts and written reports from witnesses. The jury also heard from the pharmacist who sold us Prepulsid. Among other things he testified he couldn't recall any information about the risks of Prepulsid before March 2000, and had never seen any warning like the U.S. black box warning.

At the end of the day I drove home to Oakville on the crowded QEW in deep thought, and considerable angst. The tough part was yet to come. When I opened the door, Gloria was reading some cards and admiring flowers friends and fam-ily members had sent in remembrance of Vanessa. March 19th— a flashback to one year before. It was like no time had passed. Gloria told me a woman we didn't know had called. She was very nice on the phone, explaining that her son, a friend of Vanessa, would like to visit us. Could they come over? This was puzzling as neither of us recognized his name. They arrived shortly after. Her handsome son seemed profoundly sad. He'd brought his own memorial to Vanessa—some beautiful cut flowers. I wondered if perhaps she'd been seeing this young man between classes or after school, a blooming romance we didn't know about. But it was nothing that formal. He explained that he didn't have a lot of friends. She'd been nice to him at school, stopping to say hello in the halls and talk to him. He missed her very much.

I think that was the most I had felt like Vanessa's father since she'd died. That was the Vanessa I knew. She had touched this young man's life in such a meaningful way that a year later he was inspired to honour her. Simply by chatting with him in the hall. I could picture Vanessa doing that and hear her voice in my mind. We talked a little more, and were pleased to accept his offer to keep in touch. I didn't break down until later, long after this complete stranger—a young man who had been touched by Vanessa—had left.

Day Two
Tuesday, March 20, 2001

The first doctor called as a witness was the psychiatrist who Vanessa has seen several times, most notably March 15th, three days before she collapsed. Vanessa had liked him a lot, as did I. He'd connected with her easily. His friendly manner had made her smile, and even laugh. She'd looked forward to seeing him.

Mr. O'Marra questioned him about Vanessa, if his handwritten notes about her in her medical file were correct: "no depression, no anxiety, alert, cooperative, attractive, well-groomed, 137 lbs, logical, coherent, laughed, good concentration, good memory, no suicidal intent, bulimia was under control."

"That's right," he verified.

That was the Vanessa I knew. Although Vanessa never took laxatives or diuretics and was not a binge eater—two key components of bulimia—she no doubt had a problem throwing up.

When it was Gary Will's turn, a key question he asked the doctor was: "So you had no concerns regarding the safety of Prepulsid?"

"I thought it was safe," he replied. Then, leaving no doubt, added, "My wife was on it."

On his turn, Johnson & Johnson's counsel, Mr. McKee, asked twice if Vanessa had been taking laxatives and diuretics, which can cause an electrolyte disorder. Here we go, I thought. I understood the lawyers had a responsibility to represent their clients, but this was hard to listen to.

He didn't back down: "No."

The lawyer for the doctors, asked if the doctor had any concerns that Vanessa might be at risk when he saw her March 15th.

"No," he said, and then tilted his head and gazed up as if he was remembering her. He smiled: "She was the picture of health." One for our side, I thought.

As the last doctor to see her before she collapsed his description would be strong evidence Vanessa was an otherwise healthy girl with one problem. I hoped the fact that the doctor's wife was on Prepulsid would help establish in the jury's mind that the doctors hadn't seen the five Prepulsid warning letters.

The coroner asked him how common purging was in Vanessa's peer group.

"It's hard to say," he testified. "So much is hidden. Perhaps 5 to 20 per cent."

I'd read that as many as 25 per cent of teenaged girls have a problem throwing up after meals, not exactly rare.

Each time there was a break in the proceedings the public relations man from Johnson & Johnson would zero in on any journalists in the courtroom as they headed out to make phone calls or stretch their legs, making sure they heard his angle on the latest testimony. Frankly, to obtain equal time, I did the same, filling in the blanks for stories the journalists would hand in for publication the next day. I didn't have much to do at the break.

The next witness, Dr. Stu MacLeod, was a professor of

Clinical Epidemiology and Biostatistics, Medicine, and Pediatrics at McMaster University. He'd authored more than 190 publications, and served on numerous national and international advisory committees related to his expertise in clinical pharmacology and toxicology, and, perhaps most important for our inquest—pediatric pharmacology. The coroner had requested that Dr. MacLeod explain the basics of drug toxicity to the jury, and come back another day to answer questions on this specific death. I had no idea if his testimony would help or hurt our case.

"How would you define drug toxicity?" Mr. O'Marra asked.

"Any non-beneficial effect of a drug," Dr. MacLeod replied. "Usually a modifier is added—major or minor toxicity. Every drug has some toxicity, from trivial to life threatening." With regards to drug labels he said there is "semantic confusion." "Doctors are not linguists." I hoped the jury could translate this medical-speak.

Dr. MacLeod commented on adverse drug reactions: "Adverse drug reaction reporting is very erratic. Health Canada officials are fully aware of the fact they have totally inadequate resources. They are seeing the tip of a very large iceberg."

Regarding off-label use his remarks were very revealing: "Doctors don't think in terms of off-label/on-label. They know how they can use drugs from their colleagues. No doctor accepts that Health Canada should tell them how to practice medicine. Health Canada is not on their radar screen." Dr. MacLeod would return to provide more testimony later.

I did not attend the third day of the hearing. The key evidence was to be from the pathologist who had conducted Vanessa's autopsy. By law an autopsy had been compulsory, but the whole idea made me sick at heart. But there had been a bright note that day, Gary Will explained the next morning. The pathologist testified she believed it was Prepulsid that played the major role in Vanessa death, not an electrolyte imbalance. One more for us.

Day Four
Thursday, March 22, 2001

Dr. Kayner had been Vanessa's family doctor since she was two years old. He was a hard working doctor whose waiting room was usually full. We'd found him to be an excellent diagnostician and trusted him totally. He first prescribed Prepulsid for Vanessa in 1999. She told him it helped her. He'd seen no trouble with the drug before.

"She felt bloated as a young child, I recall. This was atypical. I thought there might be a motility disorder: slow gastric emptying." So he referred Vanessa to the GE, who recommended a motility test.

"When did you first learn the results were negative?"

"After Vanessa's death."

Dr. Kayner testified he had never checked the Prepulsid label in the *CPS*. And he never saw the final Prepulsid warning letter sent out in late February until March. At that time he decided this was "like Seldane all over again" and decided to not renew any Prepulsid prescriptions and directed his assistant to do the same. Mr. O'Marra asked Dr. Kayner: "Was there anything in that warning letter that implied you should call your patients on Prepulsid and get them off it?"

"No."

As I feared, the Johnson & Johnson lawyer asked Dr. Kayner what he would have done if Vanessa was throwing up more often than she said. It was starting. I thought this would be their strategy: *Vanessa was throwing up far more than she said. Her electrolytes were imbalanced because of that. Who could have known?* It was so hard for me to sit in silence and listen him say these words in front of the jury. It was not true. The source of his question was a statement from one of Vanessa's friends in the police report who thought Vanessa's problem was worse than it was. But the doctor's records showed Vanessa had been very honest about it. It was under control. I scrutinized the faces of the people on the jury to see if his words were gaining any traction. I couldn't tell. It was nerve-wracking.

Dr. Kayner answered that he would have run a barrage of tests and taken her off Prepulsid. But, he said: "That's not the Vanessa I saw."

Gary Will questioned Dr. Kayner about his experience with the Janssen-Ortho detail rep. The rep had visited twice a year and had promoted Prepulsid, leaving glossy flyers behind, he said.

In the U.S. Janssen had disseminated brochures that promoted Prepulsid for unapproved uses in 1998. The FDA referred to them as "false and misleading" in an official rebuke sent to Janssen in June 1998.[1] But Gary Will was not allowed to talk about that in front of the jury.

However, Exhibit #29 in this inquest was a Canadian brochure, which compared Prepulsid with ranitidine.[2] On the front page it announced to doctors in large bold print: "Don't delay. Treat the underlying cause of stomach complaints right away." In slightly smaller print: "*Delayed gastric emptying may be the underlying cause for up to 60% of patients with stomach complaints.*" Delayed gastric emptying was why Dr. Kayner gave Vanessa Prepulsid. Underneath that it read: "*By treating the underlying cause, Prepulsid was more effective (than ranitidine) at relieving the full range of symptoms,*" with a bolded checkmark beside a list of symptoms: including bloating *and vomiting*.

Gary asked Dr. Kayner about the brochure: "In each case Prepulsid is ahead of ranitidine in every respect—including bloating, including vomiting. Was this consistent with their sales pitch?"

"I believe that is probably correct."

"You prescribed it because of this?"

"Partially because of the pharmaceutical reps."

"For safety, you would rely on the drug manufacturer?"

"Absolutely."

"The reps told you it was safe."

"Yes."

"It was routinely used?"

"Yes, at our hospital and [other hospitals]."

"The reps never told you to *not* prescribe it for eating disorders?"

"No. Never."

Dr. Kayner had broken down and was weeping on the stand. The coroner called a short recess.

At the end of the day something went wrong. As I was putting my coat on I overheard the lawyers from the other parties talking. They were planning where they would all meet for dinner.[3] An alarm went off for me. I told Gary what I'd heard. He said they could talk with whomever they wanted. What might they discuss over dinner? I wondered. I soon found out.

There were two ways everybody could get off the hook. First, since Vanessa was taking Prepulsid as described and nothing else, they couldn't suggest overdose or another drug taken at the same time. So they would try to persuade the jury that even though Vanessa was generally healthy, she was throwing up far more than she told her doctors, *and* that she had a hidden genetic defect—cardiac conduction defect. Either way Vanessa was at fault. In the following days the jury was to hear these theories raised *ad nauseam*, in the form of repeated leading questions.

When I arrived home that day Gloria was in distress.

She'd started a new job at the Ontario Ministry of Culture and Communications that week, commuting to Toronto on the Go Train. Gloria always chose to remember Vanessa as she was, one day at a time, without dwelling on how she died. Her day-to-day focus was on our family moving forward—Madeline and Hart. But that day on the train, reality cold-cocked her like a punch in the stomach. As she glanced up from a novel she was reading she saw Vanessa's picture all around her, as her fellow commuters silently read newspapers that were covering the inquest. The headlines shouted at her: "Heartburn Drug Focus of Inquest," "Doubts Raised about Data on Drug Reactions."

"I simply can't fathom that the people we had trusted with Vanessa's health had done anything that would kill her," she told me.

I supposed this had been inevitable. But there were journalists at the inquest every day. The publicity was going to get worse. I would be so grateful when these few weeks had passed.

There were many times I thought back to my days in the government of Ontario, when I had been involved in the drug promotion system.

As a Member of Provincial Parliament in the nineties I had benefited from Big Pharma political donations.[4] I deeply regretted that. But at the time I had no idea how risky their products could be, and how the dangers are hidden to increase profits.[5] Political contributions create debts of gratitude, just like gifts to doctors. People are people. When you treat them kindly and give them something, they feel a powerful reaction—gratitude—and it's often subconscious. I am telling you this from experience. I felt it when they lobbied me. The Big Pharma lobbyists are nice people. They have a job to do. And in most cases it includes spreading around a lot of money. They do it subtly. There is no *quid pro quo.* "Hey, if I buy you dinner at Barbarians, will you speak up to help get our drug approved for the provincial formularies?" But before you finish the last bit of your beef tenderloin, you will have heard the marvellous story of how their drug keeps patients out of the hospital and saves the taxpayers hundreds of millions. They won't mention it can increase the risk of cancer or whatever the adverse effect is, and how that will *cost* the system hundreds of millions.

Traditionally, the drug companies donate the most money to the party in power[6]—but include the opposition parties. That's in case their support is needed on a government bill, or the opposition wins the next election. It's hard for any politician to refuse to meet with someone—or tell his staff not to—who recently chatted him up at his own $250 a head fundraiser.

In 2007 all business and corporate donations to federal election campaigns were banned by the Stephen Harper government. This will no doubt help create a profound change for the better in public health policy developed in our federal parliament over time.

For lobbying government, caucus members are prioritized by rank: Prime Minister (or Premier), PM's senior staff; PM's policy advisor of health issues; Minister of Health; the Minister's policy advisor on pharma; the Minister of Finance; other high-ranking Ministers; MPs where Big Pharma factories are located; or anyone who is likely to end up in these positions. They track these moves in advance—by knowing who's hot and who's not. Follow the money. Money follows power.

As of July 2008, legislation at the federal level demands that lobbyists report and register every meeting with government decision-makers at many levels by the fifteenth day of the next month or face serious fines and possibly jail time—another key reform that will help reduce undue corporate influence at the federal level.

The pharma folks—like many big business people—also bought tables at the big annual party fundraisers for $7,000 to $12,000 each.[7] They may sponsor provincial party events and donate to the favourite charities of key politicians. Sometimes they invite elected officials to golf tournaments, or splashy events at fine hotels. I've been there and done that as an MPP. And they always talk to politicians in the language of their priorities. In 1995, my government had promised to balance the Ontario budget and create jobs. So on one golf cart ride I heard their theory of how a drug saved the government millions of dollars in hospitals by reducing broken hips, and their company was . . . creating jobs.

Provincial politicians are lobbied mainly on getting Big Pharma's new drugs on the provincial formularies and fighting off generic competition. The province of Ontario is one of the biggest single customers for drugs in North America. So getting a drug on their list is like winning a jackpot. In 2005 Ontario spent $3.5 billion on drugs, and in 2002–2003 they paid $100 million for one heartburn drug—Losec. But many company drug plans and union contracts copy the provincial formularies. So getting one new drug on the Ontario formulary could be worth hundreds of millions in sales over a few years. And that's just one province!

Federal politicians are lobbied for things like better patent protection, better tax treatment and—most importantly for you and I—changes to regulations that can endanger patients. In recent years Big Pharma has been pushing for faster drug approvals—the kind that led to hundreds of deaths in the U.S.[8] They are also working quietly behind the scenes for approval to advertise drugs directly to consumers in Canada, another risky practice that creates blockbusters.

The most effective political debts of gratitude have been created during party leadership campaigns. Corporations are no longer allowed to donate federally, but until 2007 individuals were allowed to donate $5,400 to each leadership candidate. In 2006, one candidate—Liberal Joe Volpe—actually accepted donations of $5,400 from the children of generic drug manufacturer Apotex's current and former senior managers for his leadership bid, along with their parent's money totalling

$108,000. That is obviously an inappropriate debt of gratitude related to one company. When people in leadership positions have such poor judgment, how hard can it be for Big Pharma to increase their influence? (Under media pressure Joe gave some of it back.)[9]

Big Pharma also hire former politicians and scoop current staff into highly paid senior positions to benefit from their relationships.[10] It's not just their way of saying thanks. It's about facetime with decision-makers. For example, they hired former Ontario minister of health Murray Elston as president of Rx&D, the key lobby group for the brand companies in Canada, and his former parliamentary assistant at the Ministry of Health—Chris Ward—as vice-president. Prior to that former federal minister of consumer and corporate affairs Judy Erola was president. Rx&D's latest president, Russell Williams, is a well-connected former Quebec MLA. Quebec is very special to Big Pharma because they purchase brand-name drugs for fifteen years after they are listed, even if a generic becomes available, sometimes years longer than the other provinces.[11] Sadly, this means elderly and poor Quebec residents have been forced to effectively subsidize some of the wealthiest corporations in the world out of pocket with co-payments and deductibles for high priced brand name drugs, when cheaper generics are available.

Sometimes Big Pharma hire people to lobby their former bosses. In 2004, John Duffy—good friend and former transition team member to Prime Minister Paul Martin—was hired to lobby the feds for Merck Frosst, and to help Ward Health Strategies "stop Canadian Internet pharmacies selling into the United States."[12]

This is another practice recently banned at the federal level by the Harper government. Transition-team members are forbidden by law from acting as consultant lobbyists for five years.

In the late nineties AstraZeneca hired Queen's Park ministerial staffer Sheila Frame, who then hand-picked three more

QP staffers—one out of the premier's office and two from ministers' offices—to help AstraZeneca do business at Queen's Park, when AstraZeneca was trying to get blockbuster Nexium on the Ontario formularies.

Since the 1980s Ottawa has extended the patent protection periods for brand-name drugs three times. The Mulroney government extended it from seven to twenty years in 1987 when Rx&D promised they would raise their R&D investments in Canada to 10 per cent of sales. They haven't kept that promise for the last five years.[13] Yet in September 2002 they had the nerve to promise to increase their R&D investments in Canada in exchange for—are you ready?—longer patents.[14]

When I was MPP, during one week in 1999 I received phone calls from two pharma presidents who basically reamed me out because their new drugs had been turned down for the Ontario formularies. They were furious. "Our industry supports your government. We max out our donations to your party. We are bringing in investment and jobs. And we can't even get our drugs on the formularies." The messages were almost identical, I suspect because they just came from the same meeting. I wasn't on the Executive Council (Cabinet) and hadn't even seen any official drug list, let alone had any say on what should be on it. Someone from these companies must have contacted every friendly government member to express their angst.

Does this stuff work? Does Big Pharma get what it wants?

In 2006 the Ontario McGuinty government introduced Bill 102 to save the taxpayers $300 million a year on drugs out of its total brand-name drug bill of "$2.7 billion, more than it spends on transportation, culture, and the environment combined."[15] Amongst other things Bill 102 would have made cheaper generic substitutions easier. That would cost Big Pharma some profits. So Rx&D hired Health Minister George Smitherman's former chief of staff, Jason Greer, and Premier McGuinty's former Director of Issues Management, Bob Lipinski, to convince the government that cheaper drugs were a bad idea. They got a meeting with the premier. Showing off how they exert influence on nations, Big Pharma also apparently had the British High Commissioner to Canada write a rather menacing letter to Premier McGuinty [16]

The Ontario government backed down on key clauses on Bill 102. [17]

These things were very much on my mind as the Health Canada doctor began his testimony at the inquest.

Chapter 17

Friends in Very
High Places

*"The relationship between a regulator and the regulated . . .
must never become one in which the regulator loses sight of
the principle that it regulates only in the public interest and
not in the interest of the regulated."*
—Justice Horace Krever, Commission of Inquiry on the Blood
System in Canada, 1996

*In November 2003, I received a letter from Maryann Murray in
Carlisle, Ontario, just a half-hour from Oakville. Maryann and
her husband, Paul, had lost their beautiful twenty-two-year-old
daughter Martha to an adverse drug reaction. We sat down over
coffee at a local restaurant and Maryann told me their story.
They had said goodnight to Martha on September 24, 2002 and
then found her in her bedroom the next morning, dead of a heart
attack. Three years had passed and there had been no significant changes at Health Canada. There is an unspoken bond
between parents who have lost a child, and my heart went out
to the Murrays.*

They had trusted the system and it had let them down at every step. A specialists report in Martha's medical file said to not give her lithium because it was dangerous with low potassium—a condition from which Martha suffered. She was given lithium anyway and her dosage increased thirteen days before she died. In March 2003, the local coroner reported Martha's death as "natural." But in November 2003, the Pediatric Death Review Committee of the Chief Coroner's Office reported: "Martha's use of prescribed lithium, especially in the setting of hypokalemia [low potassium] would put her at risk for a cardiac event." On November 29, 2004, I went down to the Ontario Legislative Assembly's Question Period to support the Murrays as MPP Shelly Martel requested an inquest into Martha's death. The government refused. In February 2005, an investigation statement signed by the Chief Coroner's office changed the cause of Martha's death to "unascertained."

Some time later Maryann received a letter from the coroner's office in Hamilton saying they had authorized the destruction of Martha's heart. That's one way to end an investigation.[1]

Day Six
Monday, March 26, 2001

The full inquest did not sit on Friday as the coroner heard representations from the parties regarding Janssen-Ortho documents.

On Monday the doctor from Health Canada began his testimony. He spent several hours on the stand explaining the drug regulatory process at Health Canada. Gary Will questioned him on the Canadian safety warnings on Prepulsid in January 2000, pointing out that in the U.S. the warnings were published and broadcast by the major media outlets.[2]

Q. It was important that at the time of the Dear Healthcare letter in Canada that there be a public warning that was given, that was picked up by the major media?

A. Correct.

Q. And Health Canada was insistent that there be a public warning in Canada?

A. That is correct.

Q. Janssen didn't want to give a public warning in Canada?

A. They did not initially agree to it. They subsequently did.

Q. But their initial response was that they had no intention of issuing a general public statement or advisory?

A. I believe they said that.

Q. And they said that to Health Canada?

A. Yes.

Sure enough, filmmaker Erna Buffie had obtained a copy of a letter from Janssen VP Wendy Arnott dated January 15, 2000 to Marta Caris, acting director of the Bureau of Pharmaceutical Assessment at Health Canada. It read: "Janssen-Ortho does not have the intention of issuing a 'general public statement or advisory' regarding Prepulsid to accompany the Dear Healthcare Professional letter. We are not aware of any regulatory requirement regarding the issuance of a general public statement ... We would be grateful if you would share with us the 'Departmental procedure' calling for such a document; perhaps pointing us to the appropriate location of this document on the TPP [Therapeutics Products Program] website would be most efficient."

In other words, unless you can show me an official regulation or procedure that says we must, we aren't going to issue a public warning, so stop bothering us.

When I first saw this letter, I realized the last chance to save Vanessa's life had been lost due to this decision at Janssen-Ortho.

Dr. Kayner had testified he didn't see the final warning letter until March, and then decided to not renew any prescriptions, directing his assistant to do the same. Had a warning been issued in January I believe Dr. Kayner would have seen it in February, and Vanessa would be alive. Sadly, this jury would never see that letter. But Gary promised to get these facts before the jury with questions, and he did a superb job. The doctor's testimony continued with a question from Gary Will:

Q.   And did Health Canada eventually respond to that after some time had passed that, "If you don't do it, Janssen, we're going to do it?"
A.   We, in effect, said that, yes.
Q.   And it was only when Health Canada threatened to go public themselves, that Janssen agreed to issue a public warning?
A.   They did agree.

He was avoiding the answer: a simple "yes." We also had a letter dated February 17, 2000, from Marta Caris to Janssen-Ortho VP Wendy Arnott insisting that a "balanced message be communicated to consumers. Should these not be acceptable terms to Janssen-Ortho, the Therapeutics Products Program will on behalf of Health Canada issue its own Dear Healthcare Professional letter and 'general public statement or advisory.' Please advise me by Friday, February 18th of your intentions."

That sounded like a threat to go public to me. But time had been running out. Why did Health Canada officials always seem to be beating around the bush on drug safety matters? They could have just issued a clearly worded public advisory. Then I remembered what happened to Dr. Michele Brill-Edwards.

The doctor's testimony continued with a question from Gary Will:

Q.   They agreed to a public warning but there never was a
     public warning, was there, in Canada?
A.   There was and it was released to the media.
Q.   And which of the media picked up the warning?
A.   That, I can't say.

In fact a "communications" on Prepulsid had gone out
from Janssen-Ortho dated March 2000 "in cooperation with
Health Canada." Its heading was "Revised Product Labeling
Announced for Prepulsid." Based on my experience in public
office that title almost guaranteed the media would ignore it.
His position was the same when asked about it:

A.   It would not be a message that I would want.
Q.   A better message would have been "Prepulsid could cause
     serious cardiac arrhythmias"?
A.   There should at least be a warning in my opinion.

Towards the end of his testimony Gary asked him a question that I had dreamed of asking him myself, along with key
decision-makers at Janssen-Ortho.

Q.   And for someone in the condition of Vanessa Young, if your
     children had those conditions, you wouldn't have let them
     take Prepulsid, would you?

One of the lawyers immediately objected to that question,
and the coroner ruled that the doctor wouldn't have to answer.
But it didn't matter. Everyone in the courtroom knew the answer.
He always sounded like he was a neutral observer. Everything he said would certainly protect Health Canada, but I never
once felt that he was on Vanessa's side. In fact, over the next
seven years, with the exception of Marta Caris—who sent the

threatening letter to Ms. Arnott—I never felt that anyone at the Health Canada Drugs Directorate was focused on protecting patients.

I tried one more time to assist Health Canada in November 2003 at the King Edward Hotel in Toronto. They had hired a moderator and sent a team across Canada to consult with stakeholders on "Legislative Renewal." The plan was apparently to take four old acts, including the Food and Drugs Act, and put them into one new one.[3] They even wrote a discussion paper Entitled "Health and Safety First." Translated from bureaucrat-speak by one journalist, internal Health Canada documents revealed they viewed Canada's Food and Drugs Act as "outdated because it has too narrow a focus on safety."[4]

Direct to Consumer advertising (DTC), a concern of mine, was on the agenda, so I went down to join them at the King Edward Hotel in Toronto. The participants were sitting at tables spread around the room, and once again there was a moderator at the front with a tripod and big pad of paper to write down "feedback." The day did not start well. Again there was no media present. Dr. Joel Lexchin was participating and requested that everyone declare any potential conflicts of interest. I supported this because I knew some of the participants present were registered under the name of patient advocacy groups, but pharma-funded. Some of these groups, I'd found, acted as shills for the industry, promoting their interests.

The moderator—a cheerful fellow who reminded me of a TV game show host—refused to make such a request. "Here we go again," I thought. Health Canada just didn't want to know who was getting Big Pharma money—probably because they were getting so much themselves in fees. After discussion everyone offered a "voluntary" disclosure of any funding their organization received from the pharmaceutical industry.

The safety advocates present, myself included, explained

the many reasons we felt DTC advertising was inappropriate for prescription drugs and should not be introduced.

The moderator, however, kept smiling and repeated: "I hear what you are saying, but if we did, *how* should we do it?"

Various Health Canada officials around the room were taking notes. The moderator referred to a 191-page Health Canada document he'd passed around, which contained three short paragraphs on prohibiting DTC ads, and almost six pages of suggestions *how* DTC ads might be legalized. He was steering the participants to talk about the six pages. I was convinced that day—and still am—that senior managers at Health Canada are working behind the scenes to introduce DTC advertising in Canada, despite all pretences to the contrary. This travelling dog and pony show was all about creating a document with a lot of "stakeholder" names and comments supporting exactly what Health Canada planned to do for their "partners" in the first place.

In the meanwhile the Chrétien government was acting quietly for the brand companies. In April 2003 the government replaced two of their own members on the Parliamentary Industry Committee who apparently seemed uncooperative for a crucial vote to kill an idea recommended by the Romanow Commission on Health Care—a commission created by Chrétien. The motion was to review the regulations that allowed brand-name drug companies to sue to keep cheaper generics off the market, a practice that costs Canadian patients hundreds of millions in drug costs.

A 2003 York University study proved that Canada's cheaper drug testing was putting patients at risk.[5] The study showed that our drug approval system is more like those in Europe where *drug recalls after patients are harmed are four times higher than in the U.S.* It also showed that Health Canada relies on the brand companies for advice on drug approvals, and to police advertising claims—kind of like a food inspector asking a plant manager how to inspect food.

This lack of interest in safety was expressed in the 2002 Speech from the Throne, when the federal government had begun in earnest to get out of the business of protecting Canadians. The government faced almost $12 billion in lawsuit damages for everything from faulty prescription drugs to tainted blood. Two senior bureaucrats faced criminal charges after sixty thousand Canadians had been given tainted blood—with six thousand Canadians dying as a result. It appeared the civil servants wanted to complete the transition from public protection to risk management to reduce their own personal liability as well as the government's. So they planned to revamp the Food and Drugs Act and abandon a principle of law that has protected Canadians from poisonous foods and drugs for decades—the "precautionary principle."

Precautionary principle may sound dull, but it is dynamic. It means "better safe than sorry." It's the kind of principle that requires safety checks on used cars, or has consumers examining "best before" dates on dairy products. Since thalidomide, our government has demanded that corporations prove their products are safe before they are allowed to sell them on the market. The proposed Food and Drugs Act would replace this lifesaving principle with smart regulation—a euphemism for risk management—"better sorry than safe."[6]

Health Canada's actions—or lack of action—did not go unnoticed. In April 2004 the Parliamentary Standing Committee on Health raked Health Canada over the coals for too much secrecy, for protecting Big Pharma "commercial interests" and for not effectively protecting Canadians who take prescription drugs.[7]

And a month later journalists were fed up with the shenanigans at Health Canada and awarded them the Code of Silence

Award for being Canada's most secretive government department. It was for refusing to release information on adverse drug
reactions in a useful format, and denying access to information
on prescription drugs that could harm or kill Canadians.[8]

Based on my experience in government, Health Canada
was deeply conflicted and therefore incapable of protecting
Canadians from risky drugs. Although these events occurred
after the inquest, this was the same organization we faced at the
inquest and in our civil case.

Day Seven
Tuesday, March 27, 2001

Next to testify was the internist on call when they brought
Vanessa to the hospital after her collapse. She was also the
specialist to whom Vanessa was referred by Dr. Kayner, who
sent her for a motility test two months before she died, and who
didn't remember Vanessa or me the night Vanessa collapsed. The
jury heard our doctor's credentials as a dual specialist in gastroenterology and internal medicine, that she had published papers in the area of gastroenterology, and had received the
Janssen-Ortho Motility Fellowship Award in 1998, money she
won on a competitive basis.

She was on the stand for hours and testified she was inti-
mately familiar with Prepulsid, a drug she prescribed. After seeing Vanessa back on January 19, 2000, regarding her problem
throwing up, like Dr. Kayner she felt Vanessa's problem might be
an underlying motility disorder.

The opposition theory of a cardiac conduction defect as the
cause of death was fully developed in front of the jury during the
doctor's testimony under questions from Johnson & Johnson's
lawyer:

Q. And if she had a conduction defect, it [an electrocardio-
    gram] might, although not certainly as I understand it, it
    might have shown whether she had a conduction defect?
A. It, it may show it, yes.
Q. But we don't have a fair ECG, so we just don't know
    whether she had a conduction defect or not?
A. That's correct.
Q. As I understand it, both a conduction defect and an elec-
    trolyte imbalance on their own without any medication can
    cause arrhythmia and cardiac arrest, is that right?

I glanced past him at the jury, worried that repeating the
term "conduction defect" over and over would sink into their
subconscious. They were being very attentive.

The counsel for the doctors went a step further:

Q. We've all heard the stories in the newspaper and the media
    of athletes, professional athletes who die suddenly?
A. Hm-mm, yes.
Q. Without any history of cardiac arrhythmia?
A. Yes.
Q. And would it be fair to say in an autopsy, there would be
    no pathological findings which would be consistent with
    some of the potential causes of cardiac arrhythmia which
    you describe?
A. That is quite likely, yes.
Q. Much has been made of the cisapride, Doctor. Given the
    other potential causes of cardiac arrhythmia, is it possible
    that the ingestion of the cisapride in Vanessa Young was
    nothing more that a coincidence in relation to her death?
A. It is possible.

This was painful to listen to. He got her to say that was

there would be no evidence if some invented conduction defect caused Vanessa's death. So the jury should conclude the cause of death wasn't what all the evidence pointed to. It was something that anyone might have, for which there was no evidence, and could never be any evidence.

If the invented heart conduction defect story didn't work on the jury, the backup theory—a previous electrolyte imbalance—might. The doctor testified how Vanessa appeared in January when she diagnosed her: "She was well-hydrated, well-nourished, shows no signs of any problems and she also says that on cisapride she's vomiting less. So in fact she was minimal, vomiting minimally." This was the third doctor the jury heard testify that Vanessa was otherwise a healthy girl, with a mild form of bulimia that was under control.

But the lawyers kept up the "electrolyte imbalance" theory even when shot down by friendly witnesses. For example, he asked her:

Q. And after you examined her [Vanessa] would you agree with me that it was unclear to you what caused arrhythmia or arrest at that time?

A. Yes.

Q. The possibilities included a pre-existent cardiac conduction defect of the heart?

A. That is most certainly the case.

Q. And from what you said earlier in your testimony I take it an electrolyte imbalance is also a possibility as a cause of arrhythmia?

A. Well, certainly we do not know what her potassium or what her other electrolytes would have been at the time of arrest.

Shot down on the electrolyte imbalance theory. If true,

Prepulsid would have been contraindicated for Vanessa. She stuck with the conduction defect theory. If it was true, it would make her lack of warning to Vanessa about Prepulsid irrelevant.

The doctor testified that she met with the Janssen drug rep but never discussed safety. And she had prescribed Prepulsid widely for years. After seeing Vanessa on January 19, 2000, she prescribed a motility test for February 4, 2000, at McMaster University Medical Centre in Hamilton. I accompanied Vanessa. The test results had never come back and she did not follow up. The jury heard that her office didn't even ask about the results until March 1, 2000, when I called Dr. Kayner's office and asked where they were.

Then it appeared that our doctor had told the coroner and all the lawyers at an off-record conference before the proceedings that morning that in her opinion Vanessa's electrolytes were at a normal (safe) level when she collapsed. Gary Will questioned her about this on the stand.

Q.   And is it your personal opinion that her electrolyte readings at the time of arrest [her collapse] were also within normal limits?

The doctor replied in various ways that she could not speculate and no one could say. There was a private conference of the lawyers with the coroner at the front, and Gary tried again. He asked, or tried to ask, the same question four times:

Q.   Prior to 9:30 this morning did you have an opinion as to the probable level of her electrolytes prior to arrest?
A.   Yes.
Q.   And was it your opinion at that time that her electrolytes were within normal limits prior to arrest?
A.   I really could not tell. I think it could go either way.

Q. Did you state to your counsel that it was more likely than
    not that her electrolytes were within normal limits prior to
    Vanessa Young's arrest?

Coroner: Please don't answer that question.

Some more off-the-record discussion took place. Gary Will
tried again:

Q. I go back to my point of what was told to counsel about
    this witness's evidence . . . Did you express an opinion in a
    boardroom where I was present, [doctor's counsel] was
    present, and all counsel were present, that it was your per-
    sonal opinion that Vanessa Young's electrolytes prior to ar-
    rest would have been within normal limits?

Gary asked eight more questions attempting—unsuccess-
fully—to get her to repeat what she had allegedly said in front
of the coroner and all the other lawyers in the boardroom before
9:30 that same morning.

The jury also heard from the doctor's written report to Dr.
Kayner on January 19, 2000: "If she [Vanessa] does have an
abnormal gastric emptying time, I will encourage her to stay on
the Prepulsid and look for causes of gastroparesis. If, however,
she has normal emptying time, *then I will concentrate in
behaviour modification with her*." [my italics] Here is an exchange between Gary Will, the coroner and our doctor on why
she did not direct Dr. Kayner to take Vanessa off Prepulsid.

Q. Doctor, when you met with Vanessa in January was it not
    your intention if gastroparesis was ruled out, that the
    Prepulsid would stop?

A. My intention at that time was that she should go to behav-
    ioural therapy; cognitive, no, behavioural therapy to help

her with her eating problems.

Coroner: I didn't hear any answer to that. Could you repeat the question please, Mr. Will?

Q.   Was it your intention in January of 2000 that once gastro-paresis was ruled out, to take Vanessa off Prepulsid?

A.   That would not be . . . My main concern is that if gastro-paresis was ruled out, that she has behaviour modification.

She was the expert. We'd all heard that when the test ruled out gastroparesis, she never contacted Dr. Kayner. *Was there was any reason for Vanessa to be taking Prepulsid?* Was this another missed opportunity to avert her death?

Coroner: I'm still not hearing an answer to the question. The question is: a negative test result would have resulted in you taking her off the cisapride?

A.   That would be a judgment call. She keeps telling us that she, when she takes Prepulsid, she vomits less.

Gary's face had slowly gone red, but his voice never changed pitch, and he never appeared agitated. He tried to get an answer another way.

Q.   Doctor, you were trying to determine whether she had gas-troparesis in order to determine whether she still needed Prepulsid?

A.   That is putting the question too simply. My job is to help her and you know, I wanted to make sure she doesn't have gastroparesis and therefore, you know, rule that problem out, make the proper diagnosis so that she could have treat-ment. And if the diagnosis turns out to be a behaviour problem, then she should have behaviour modification.

Q.   And that behaviour modification wouldn't include taking Prepulsid, would it?

A. Probably not. That would be up to the psychologist treating her.

You have to give Gary credit. He didn't give up. I hoped the jury was thinking what I was: What is this witness hiding? And why would an expert on the digestive system, who had just proved with a test that a drug that was risky for anyone throwing up was not needed, allow a psychologist to decide if that risky drug should be continued?

But the jury had already heard what evidence there was of any conduction heart defect in Vanessa's heart from the GE:

Q. [Gary Will] So there isn't any evidence of any conduction defect, is that right?
A. We, no.
Q. And you examined Vanessa and took a medical history and there wasn't anything in that history that raised any concern of any cardiac problem?
A. No.
Q. There wasn't a family history of a cardiac problem?
A. No.
Q. There wasn't a personal history of a cardiac problem?
A. No.
Q. And there wasn't any evidence in terms of what you saw or in any of the tests that were performed that showed any cardiac problem?
A. No.

One for our side. In the seventies, if a Ford Pinto burst into flames after being rear-ended, they didn't spend a lot of time looking for careless smoking. I watched the jury during the doctor's testimony. There was no clue what its thoughts might be.

But there was a problem with the jury. The coroner had

excused one of the jurors—a woman—due to illness. If the remaining four disagreed on a finding, two on each side, they could potentially be deadlocked on any issue. I felt our case would be much better received by a woman, especially if she was a mother. I'd just lost a sympathetic juror. This I felt could only hurt our chances.

Research grants are viewed as an honour, and are important to medical careers. Before sitting down Gary Will asked her how much money she received in 1998 for the Janssen-Ortho Motility Fellowship Award. She replied she didn't know—the money went to a supervisor. I later learned she had received $42,000 in salary from that award to do whatever she wanted to further her research and career. I felt it was very odd that a doctor could receive a financial award, and not know how much it was for.

Alan Cassels had told me the drug companies control most research by controlling what is studied. And they influence every organization that influences prescription drugs—including governments. Alex Demerse said they usually get what they want in Washington and Ottawa. But in 2002, U.S. senator Richard J. Durbin (D. Ill.) went further, saying "PhRMA, this lobby has a death grip on Congress."

My research showed that by any measure Big Pharma influence on public policy is greater in the U.S. By 2005 Big Pharma had set a new U.S. record for spending on lobbying costs over seven years: $675 million.[9] They had hired over three thousand lobbyists—over *a third of them former federal officials.*

But I was shocked to learn about the full influence Big Pharma wields on government policy in Canada—programmed from head offices in Europe and the U.S.

In 2003 I came across a story written from confidential documents that had been leaked to the *New York Times*, outlining how the key Big Pharma lobby group PhRMA planned to spend $1 million in Canada "to change the Canadian healthcare system" and $450,000 to stem the flow of low-price prescription drugs from online pharmacies in Canada to customers in the United States.

I don't know about you, but when international drug companies secretly plan to "change" the healthcare system of my sovereign nation to meet their own ends, I tend to fight back. If there was any better proof these international corporations should not be considered to be our partners in health, this was it.

But in 2004 the true scope of Big Pharma's political power was demonstrated in a way that was more like a Hollywood comedy than real life. When Big Pharma says jump, some world leaders say how high. And sometimes it's downright embarrassing. In 2004 Big Pharma lobbyists had President Bush and Prime Minister Paul Martin fussed over a bunch of Canadian pharmacies that were selling prescription drugs over the Internet— mostly to American seniors. Their crime? Selling them at Canadian prices.[10] And it wasn't as if the supporters of cheaper drugs were a bunch of liberal troublemakers trying to bring down America. One was Michael Bloomberg—billionaire Republican mayor of New York City, hoping to shave $108 million off from the city's employee drug plan![11]

The scary stories planted in the media to frighten U.S. seniors got more ridiculous as time passed. It was like the Keystone Kops. First they claimed the drugs from Canada were not the same and could be dangerous. The drugs are exactly the same drugs, usually made in the exact same factory.[12] So that fizzled. Then, they played the terrorism card. They actually claimed Internet pharmacies in Canada were funding terrorism.[13] Presidential hopeful Rudy Giuliani got involved—doing an imaginative presentation on the subject for a U.S. Senate Sub-Committee. Finally, PhRMA got caught commissioning a fictitious book in which an attack on the U.S. would be carried out by a Canadian Internet pharmacy: *The Karasik Conspiracy*.[14] The official denial from PhRMA said their senior management knew nothing about it: a renegade employee acted on his own. Kind of a "lone bookman" theory.

Since American consumers were apparently too smart, the PR spin doctors turned up the heat on the Canadians. They claimed Canada might run out of drugs! This is less likely than Canada running out of new cars. Because if the brand companies couldn't supply drugs to Canadians, our government would immediately give the job to a generic drugmaker by compulsory license. But fear works, especially when you get local politicians involved.

In anticipation of President G.W. Bush's visit to Canada in November 2004 Canadian Minister of Health Ujjal Dosanjh went down to the Harvard Medical School in Boston and warned Americans if the Internet drug business keeps growing he might try and stop the shipments from Canada. "We certainly cannot be the drugstore for the United States of America."[15] In questioning he admitted that Canadians hadn't encountered any drug shortages thus far. After the President's visit Dosanjh admitted to CTV news that U.S. President George Bush had raised the matter with Prime Minister Paul Martin.[16]

Then Minister Dosanjh began preaching that Canada might run out of drugs; telling reporters we need to protect the drug supply, and he was extremely worried, despite admitting again his department had no hard evidence that online druggists had caused shortages of drugs in Canada.

There were also rumours that the drug companies would stop selling their drugs in Canada. GlaxoSmithKline threatened to stop selling to retailers and wholesalers in Canada. They frightened some seniors I'm sure, until it backfired—consumer groups picketed their Philadelphia headquarters and threatened to boycott their products. I believe it was all bravado. The Internet is just another distribution channel for their highly profitable products. I don't think a sales-driven company making huge profits would really walk away from its eighth-largest market, Canada. Instead, Canadians can look forward to further stealthy attempts by these international companies to influence our governments.

Chapter 18

You Must Be Sick . . . Because They Need You to Be

"Formerly, when religion was strong and science weak, men mistook magic for medicine; now when science is strong and religion weak; men mistake medicine for magic."
—Thomas Szasz

Day Nine
Thursday, March 29, 2001

UNDER QUESTIONING FROM David Carruthers, assistant Coroner's Counsel, the Health Canada doctor continued his testimony from Monday, providing a detailed description of the drug approval process, and the five warning letters that went out to doctors in Canada about Prepulsid. He also explained there were a number of patients—about 150—who had life-threatening neurological impairment or severe gastroparesis for whom the risks of Prepulsid were clearly acceptable, if managed safely.

Unfortunately for us, the jury also heard more inference that Vanessa had misled her doctors. Acting for the doctors, Mr. Lerner described Vanessa's "clinical picture" and asked him:

Q. Given that clinical picture, would you agree with me, Doctor, that it would be reasonable therapeutic judgment in mid-February, 2000, to prescribe cisapride?

A. Using those parameters, I cannot see any contraindication described in those parameters. [sic]

Q. And let me add one more factor in it. The patient denied vomiting.

A. Correct.

Q. The same answer?

A. Yes.

Q. Thank you doctor.

A minute later the Johnson & Johnson lawyer asked him:

Q. Good afternoon, Doctor. Just following up on a point [defense counsel] made. Is it fair to say that a fifteen-year-old young woman can look the picture of health and is suffering from bulimia but still have an electrolyte problem?

A. I'm not an expert in bulimia, but from my reading I understand that can occur. But I am not an expert in bulimia.

Q. Are you expert enough to say that people can have electrolyte problems and still look the picture of health on the outside, ignoring the bulimia?

A. There . . . I'm not an expert in fluid and electrolyte disturbance, so I really can't comment.

Clearly that wasn't the answer the opposition wanted to hear, but I feared they were making headway with the jury anyway, raising electrolyte disorders and conduction heart defect day after day. I prayed they remembered Dr. Kayner's words: "She looked very well—a healthy, robust female every time I saw her," which were very similar to the psychiatrists: "the picture of perfect health." Our GE's records also showed that Vanessa had no visible signs of any problem.

And the coroner had explained to the jury that *answers are evidence*; questions are not evidence. But how could the repeated questions not get into the jury's subconscious?

Gary Will questioned him about a 1992 report from the World Health Organization on Prepulsid that showed it was associated with cardiac arrhythmias, and asked if Janssen had ever brought it to Health Canada's attention. I was surprised to hear he'd never heard of it. The jury also heard that there was nothing in Canada to prevent Janssen-Ortho from issuing the same kind of warning as they had in the U.S.

Days Ten and Eleven
Friday, March 30, and Monday, April 2, 2001

Wendy Arnott was vice-president of Regulatory Quality, Medical and Linguistics at Janssen-Ortho Inc., the person at Janssen in charge of issuing safety warnings in Canada. She represented Johnson & Johnson at the inquest and was on the stand for more than two days. It was Ms. Arnott's email exchange with Marta Caris at Health Canada that had been exposed by filmmaker Erna Buffie's Freedom of Information request.

By this time I felt the most important factor in our tragedy was the decision at Janssen-Ortho to not provide Canadians with the same warning for Prepulsid, similar to the 1998 U.S. black box warning adopted in 1998. Yet Ms. Arnott testified that she would not regularly keep informed about the regulatory status of Prepulsid in the U.S.[1] Monitoring FDA actions, she said, was not part of her job. That was done out of the Janssen

Research Foundation in Belgium, she testified.[2] And the Canadian data on serious ADRs was "meaningless" because our population was too small.[3]

Yet Ms. Arnott also testified that product monographs (labels) provide Canadian physicians with "accurate and complete prescribing information to use"[4]—labels that included only *adverse reactions experienced by Canadians*. Doctors believed the risk information on the label was accurate and complete, including serious reactions. Ms. Arnott knew it was meaningless.

So Health Canada relies on a private company based on another continent, with a conflicting commercial interest, to collect and monitor deadly adverse reactions from drugs we take—but they only publish in Canada the deadly reactions that occur in Canada.

Gary Will tried to determine how many people had actually died in relation to Prepulsid worldwide from Ms. Arnott, something that I've still found impossible to determine seven years later. He asked Ms. Arnott if Janssen-Ortho Inc. in Canada had access to the global database of Spontaneous Adverse Reaction Reports, residing at Janssen Research Foundation in Belgium.[5] The answer was no. They feed into it, but can't view it.

I was shaken. That sounded like a chain of convenience stores reporting sales figures or "shrinkage" to head office, but no one there providing the crucial feedback to the store managers.

Ms. Arnott said they had to send a question to the head office people in Belgium, who would query the global database and provide an answer. Then, as I sat in utter amazement, the jury got a glimpse of how much Wendy Arnott, the person at Janssen who had personally "negotiated" and delayed the final warning for Prepulsid in Canada, knew about adverse reactions from Prepulsid. Gary asked if she knew how many cardiac arrhythmias and deaths were associated with Prepulsid worldwide in September 1998. No, she didn't. She said that it was not realistic to expect her to have specific numbers. But she could get that information.

The inquest then broke for lunch while Ms. Arnott went off to call head office in Belgium. Wendy Arnott was the highest-ranking person that Health Canada officials and our doctors relied on for honest, accurate, up-to-date safety information about Johnson & Johnson drugs. And she was giving sworn testimony to help prevent more tragedies from adverse reactions. Yet her answer had revealed that she didn't know how many injuries and deaths were officially associated with Prepulsid worldwide in 1998—nor could she know how many to date. *Because Janssen Research Foundation kept that information secret.* Based on the comments I'd read in the interview with Janssen founder Dr. Paul Janssen, this didn't surprise me: "Today for the slightest thing going wrong patients go and see a lawyer." To my mind Ms. Arnott's answer revealed that either she had no access to those numbers, she didn't ask for them before coming to the inquest, or she chose not to know them. Or perhaps all three. And it verified that probably no one in Canada knew the true number of Prepulsid-related deaths worldwide. What an illusion of safety Canadian doctors and patients are under.

I joined Gary Will and his associate Chris Morrison for lunch, as we'd done many days, down the block at Fingers Bar and Grill. Friday was the big go-to-lunch day in Hamilton, and Fingers was lively with office workers talking, laughing, eating, and smoking. I asked Gary how we were doing.

He was in deep thought, and raised his eyebrows. "It's very surprising that the Canadian division of Janssen didn't track the worldwide numbers of adverse reactions and deaths in Canada."

"Well it's after 6 p.m. in Belgium," I said. "How will Wendy Arnott reach anyone at head office now?"

"I wonder," he said. "It'll be interesting to see what we hear after lunch—about the total number of deaths."

I asked Gary about the warnings, which would be key to our civil case.

"The jury's heard from two of Vanessa's doctors. They didn't see any warning letters before the last one in March. [The child psychiatrist] wouldn't have allowed his wife to take Prepulsid if he had. And I hope they picked up that Janssen refused to issue a public warning in January when Health Canada initially directed them to."

"But what about the cause of death?" I asked.

"It's hard to say with [the doctor's] testimony. She supported their conduction defect theory. But will the jury find her credible? Having to be asked the same question repeatedly doesn't help. They might have found her evasive."

"Might have?" I said. "You had to ask fifteen times about what she had said to the coroner and lawyers that morning concerning Vanessa's electrolyte levels at the time of her collapse," I said, "I counted."

Gary smiled knowingly and raised his eyebrows. "I didn't realize it was that many times." I couldn't help smiling as well.

As the waiter set our lunches down on the table Gary got serious again: "Your testimony will be important."

When the inquest resumed, Ms. Arnott continued her testimony. Remarkably, she was lucky enough to get someone in Belgium on the phone after normal business hours who could access the worldwide database. Janssen's official number of deaths worldwide related to Prepulsid as of February 28, 2000, was eighty-eight, with 353 serious arrhythmias. Their numbers just kept on growing. But Janssen's number was still well below the number of deaths Public Citizen had written about to the FDA, 106, and the number published in the L.A. Times, 302. What was the true number worldwide? How I wished I could have told the jury about the seven out of nine deaths at Joseph Brant Hospital. But that evidence had been ruled out.

Despite her lack of knowledge about the number of deaths

worldwide from Prepulsid, Ms. Arnott had been well prepared to describe Johnson & Johnson's warm relationship with Health Canada based on "mutual respect and trust." I wrote this down when she said it and will never forget it: ". . . we treat Health Canada as a customer, and a key customer of ours."[6] I found this very unsettling. Their "key customer" was the government agency who wouldn't even talk about Sana's Prepulsid report. In seven years I never got better insight into why so many drug injuries are officially tolerated in Canada. The tail is wagging the dog. Imagine if American Airlines claimed that Canada's National Transportation Safety Board—the board that investigates air crashes—was their key customer! If Health Canada is Johnson & Johnson's key customer, who is looking out for our families?

At the end of each day I'd drive back to Oakville on the QEW, reviewing key evidence in my mind. So far I'd filled three writing pads with detailed notes and quotations. And late into the evenings and on weekends I'd sift through the pages carefully looking for statements I felt would hurt our case or were outright wrong—to refute later. The remaining four jurors had heard a lot of conflicting testimony, much of it in medical-speak. For the opposition, confusion was almost as good as convincing the jury—muddy the waters. We were the ones who had to prove something—Prepulsid caused Vanessa's death—and we needed to disprove two negatives: Vanessa had no conduction defect, and she had no electrolyte disorder. The other side could win by planting seeds of doubt.

Yet failure was unthinkable. Gary Will and Chris Morrison who joined our team later that week were doing a superb job. Gary said my testimony would be important. But Gary understated things. I knew it would be critical. Late at night I wrote down all the things I would say to the jury—if the coroner would let me. Things that would convince those four people that Vanessa was an innocent victim of a dangerous drug. Obsessed wasn't a strong enough word to describe my efforts. I was utterly absorbed. Gloria and Hart were carrying on with work and school. I wasn't providing much support for them. It would be over soon, I thought.

I was also tired. My client work was more demanding and the best way to meet potential new clients was networking at events. The night before I'd joined over 800 people at the Canadian War Plane Heritage Museum in Hamilton at a fundraising dinner for a rising star MPP, Brad Clark, who was a great help to one of my clients, St. Peter's Hospital. It was so strange to be socializing and handing out business cards in the evenings, and walking through the metal detector at the John Sopinka Courthouse each morning to head upstairs and hear the grim testimony. This was my life.

Janssen VP Wendy Arnott completed her testimony on Monday. As I walked up the steps and entered our house late Monday afternoon, our golden retriever, Romulus, and our whippet, Persephone, came to greet me, tails wagging enthusiastically. I leaned over to pet them as Vanessa loved to do and glanced around, realizing that soon we'd have to sell this house we'd lived in for sixteen years. It had too many memories.

Day Twelve
Tuesday, April 3, 2001

To remind the reader, Dr. Kayner had referred Vanessa to a psychiatrist in February 1999, who was supposed to advise if there was a psychiatric component to Vanessa's symptoms. This referral had come before the meeting with the child psychiatrist. The psychiatrist had seen Vanessa only once more than a year before. In her testimony, she speculated about our family, and what Vanessa might have told her friends. She referred to Vanessa as "extremely angry" with "very poor eye contact." I was astounded. Vanessa had been described in *Oakville Today* as a gentle soul.

When I got home that evening I told Gloria what the doctor had said. Gloria and Vanessa had arrived twenty minutes late for the appointment, and the receptionist apparently had scolded them. Gloria said Vanessa had naturally felt unwelcome and upset because of this treatment.

The doctor testified that Vanessa "was extremely abrupt, and basically at that point I realized that there was no point in pursuing a history with her, because she wasn't going to give me any information." Whoa. A light went on for me: this doctor took no patient history!

It turned out that the doctor herself took no patient history. This was news to me but apparently it is not uncommon. Basically, patient history workups are subcontracted to other health care professionals—such as occupational therapists. The doctor described the process to the jury thus: the therapist screened individuals "to get a sense of the severity of the illness . . . to sort of gather the background information for me so that I could focus on the psychological aspects of it." I remembered Vanessa had attended one of these screenings on February 11, 1999, and was told by the OT she had to join a "group" to talk about her problem. She'd told me she really didn't even know what her problem was, so how could she talk about it?

"Thank God my testimony is coming up," I said to Gloria. "I'll have a chance to undo the damage to Vanessa's reputation." Understandably this gave neither of us any comfort. I continued, "You know, deep down, I guess I've been hoping that any day now one of the doctors will get on the stand and say 'We all failed her. We are all responsible. We should have done better. We are so sorry.'"

That never happened.

Day Thirteen
Wednesday, April 4, 2001[9]

Dr. Stu MacLeod returned to testify about long QT and Prepulsid. His clear statements on what caused Vanessa's death lifted my spirits. He said that the effects of cisapride on QT prolongation were well known in medical literature, and that he'd known of cisapride's effects on the QT interval for at least seven years. There is no doubt prolonged QT can lead to sudden cardiac death although it is a rare event. Although vomiting would be a causative factor, there was a *high probability* that the cause of death was cisapride.

The lawyers from the other side immediately knew they had a problem. This was the witness invited by the coroner. His resumé was unimpeachable, and testimony authoritative. The doctor's lawyer acting for the doctors, tried to get Dr. MacLeod to agree that cisapride combined with an unknown co-factor—like a cardiac abnormality—was the likely cause of death.

Dr. MacLeod said no, although an unknown co-factor could not be ruled out, he didn't believe this was the case. Consel then attempted to summarize all the possible causes of Vanessa's death in relation to cisapride:

1. Cisapride had no effect.
2. An undetected congenital problem with her heart.
3. Cisapride with a significant co-factor.

Dr. MacLeod agreed none of them could be ruled out.

I panicked. It was a trap. If those were the only possibilities, cisapride was mostly off the hook. I took a fleeting look at the jury to see if they realized it. Their faces were blank. For a brief moment I considered interrupting the proceedings to speak out. Everyone would understand. The grieving father momentarily lost control. But that would have been a tremendous mistake, damaging my own credibility and testimony. I sat silent for what seemed like forever. What should I do?

"There's one other possibility," Dr. MacLeod finally said, quietly but firmly. I closed my eyes.

"Cisapride did it alone."

I could have cheered.

By the end of the third week media attention had waned and at a break that afternoon the lone journalist in the lobby was Howard Mozel from the *Oakville Beaver*. Howard had been there almost every day, and in my view had done a good job of covering the story and getting it right in our community paper.

As I watched the Johnson & Johnson public relations man approach Howard to offer his spin, I reflected on what I was up against. This wasn't the *New York Times*, or even the *Globe and Mail*. Johnson & Johnson really left no stone unturned in influencing anything their customers and investors might read about their products and drug division Janssen-Ortho that might hurt sales or share value, even if it was sending someone to be at this inquest for every break to spin the story to the *Oakville Beaver*.

If only they did that for potentially lifesaving warnings.

When Howard was alone again I chatted with him. He hadn't missed Dr. MacLeod's one other possibility—cisapride alone.

Day Fourteen
Friday, April 6, 2001

Unfortunately, I was sure the jury would find Johnson & Johnson's expert witness, Dr. George Klein, a better and more credible witness than the GE. He was the chair of the Cardiology Division at Ontario's Western University and director of the arrhythmia service there. He was an active researcher at the university hospital in London, Ontario, and a professor who'd specialized in

290 YOU MUST BE SICK . . .

arrhythmology since 1985.

I suspected the jury members would view him as equally credible to Dr. Stuart MacLeod. The opposition apparently brought him in to expound their pre-existing conduction defect theory, which he did enthusiastically. I should mention that like Dr. MacLeod, he had never seen Vanessa, and had no firsthand personal or professional knowledge of her health. But apparently that didn't matter. Because according to Dr. Klein, anyone could fall down dead at any time with no warning. He pointed to the young coroner's constable in the court as an example. A few people in the court chuckled. Although he stated that Vanessa's cause of death was a "best guess" at best, since most people who die of sudden death have an electrical disorder in their heart, it was highly probable that Vanessa did as well. Without that—and throwing up—she would not have died. He added that if a person had a previously undetected heart defect or electrolyte imbalance a post-mortem examination would not prove it. So there would be no evidence. In Vanessa's case, there wasn't any. For Johnson & Johnson and the doctors, Dr. Klein was just what the doctor ordered.

I was watching the jury as he spoke. They were paying rapt attention. When Gary Will's chance came, he asked Dr. Klein if a family history of heart problems made the possibility of a heart problem more likely in a case of sudden death. He said yes it did. There is no history of heart arrhythmia in our family, so Gary asked him if there was *no* family history of heart arrhythmia, did it make a heart problem a less likely cause of death? He said no: family history, if not positive, does not tell you anything.

This was bizarre. If family history was relevant in helping to establish that a genetic link might make a cardiac conduction defect more likely, the fact that there was no such history or link should make a cardiac conduction defect less likely. It was either relevant or it wasn't. You don't just omit evidence when it doesn't fit your theory.

I was profoundly concerned that Dr. Klein had the last word before the jury—*after* Dr. Stuart MacLeod. The last word can be more memorable. I concluded their decision on cause of death would probably depend on whether they believed Dr. MacLeod, who said there was a high probability that cisapride was the primary cause of death, or Dr. Klein, who felt it was highly improbable. The Crown Attorney, Mr. O'Marra, apparently recognized how difficult it would be for the jury to decide, given two experts with opposing views. Upon further questioning by Mr. O'Marra, Dr. Klein said he could not eliminate the possibility that cisapride alone had caused Vanessa's death. Would it help? Who could tell?

I was cheered later that day when I got home and saw the headline in the *Oakville Beaver* written two days before: "Toxicologist Says Drug Played Role in Teen's Death." Howard Mozel at the *Oakville Beaver* hadn't missed the key point of Dr. MacLeod's testimony. I prayed the jury would be as wise.

Gloria told me Madeline had called from Queen's University, incensed. She'd just seen the psychiatrist's comment in the *Toronto Star* about Vanessa "storming" out of her office.

"That is absolute nonsense. There is no way Vanessa would ever do that." she said. That was from a sister who shared a room with Vanessa for nine years, and knew her like no one else.

Sunday was Vanessa's birthday—April 8th. She would have been seventeen. Occasionally Gloria and I had run into her friend's parents around town and heard how her friends were doing. Some were already planning which university or college to attend after finishing grade twelve next year. In my mind Vanessa was still in grade ten, still fifteen. A portion of our lives had simply stood still. We'd had a much richer life with Vanessa in it, and were grateful for those years, but would not be able to celebrate her birthday for a long time to come.

Chapter 19

There's No Such Thing as Monsters

"You see what power is—holding someone else's fear in your hand and showing it to them!"
—Amy Tan, U.S. novelist (1952–)

LATE ONE NIGHT I REFLECTED on the PR guy spinning the journalists at the inquest, and the drug industry's influence on the media. Prepulsid had been promoted to doctors for use when it wasn't proven safe. The jury had seen a brochure doing exactly that, with a checkmark beside "vomiting." And every time I turned on TV to watch the news I saw slick drug ads, like the people singing "Good Morning" and dancing in the streets for Viagra. How strong was the connection between Big Pharma and the media?

Alan Cassels had introduced me to Barbara Mintzes, a researcher at UBC, who had spent a great deal of time studying how Big Pharma promoted their drugs. I spoke with Barbara over the phone, connected by email, and chatted in person numerous times. I asked Barbara why direct-to-consumer advertising was illegal in Canada.

294 THERE'S NO SUCH THING AS MONSTERS

"Health protection," she said. "Prescription drugs that treat serious diseases are more toxic, and have less-understood risks and benefits than over-the-counter drugs. So they are only available through a doctor. Canada forbids advertising as part of that protection, as does every other country in the world—except the U.S. and New Zealand. It's because people with a debilitating illnesses or in pain are vulnerable to emotional appeals and exaggerated messages. So are their family members."

"What about the ads on TV now?" I asked

"You're seeing ads on U.S. TV channels, or Canadian 'help-seeking' ads. Our Food and Drugs Act was amended in 1978 to allow advertising only of name, price, and quantity. Health Canada has interpreted that to allow the pharma companies to advertise the indication (use) of the drug without the name. So we get the ads about diseases and conditions that raise fear and other emotions and say 'Ask your doctor. Ask your doctor.'"

"Do help-seeking ads work?"

"Yes. Very well. The pharmaceutical companies get $1.69 in new sales for every dollar spent on TV ads, and over $2 for every dollar spent on magazine ads. Our research found that three out of four doctors will give a patient a drug if they ask for it by name. But *almost as many* will get the drug if they just mention a drug ad they've seen. The doctors fill in the blanks."

"Don't people realize they're being manipulated?"

"Help-seeking ads look like public service messages. That lowers people's commercial guard. And sometimes they are broadcast or published under the auspices of a trusted patient interest group—the third-party technique—'caring people looking out for your welfare.'"

"The help-seeking ads I've seen never mention adverse reactions."

"That's right. Drugs are presented as if they are magic and work all the time, with no hint of side effects. By law U.S. DTC ads *must* mention potential side effects. Since the Canadian ads don't mention a drug, or even a drug company, they don't have to. In theory the doctors are supposed to do that." I knew how well that worked.

"We didn't know Prepulsid had serious risks. Neither did four doctors that saw Vanessa."

"That's no surprise. Studies that have been done in four countries show that detail reps almost always gave doctors the name, generic name, and indications, but not the safety information. And contraindications were never mentioned."

"The U.S. ads I've seen present the positive messages visually, while in the background a monotone voice reads a list of possible side effects."

"That's the pattern. The ads use visual images and emotion to engage the viewer, like joy, people dancing in the street for Viagra. Or guilt: in 1996 Wyeth-Ayers promised in newspaper ads that life will get better for family members too if a depressed parent seeks help—'I got my mommy back.' They also present pills as a magic way to fix complex emotional and relationship problems. Depression is explained in advertising materials as too many or too few neurotransmitter chemicals in the brain, which can of course be adjusted with an antidepressant drug. Nowhere do they mention or even imply that depression is a common human reaction to grief, loss, or other problems that might improve over time."

"Do viewers even absorb the information on side effects?"

"Sometimes. But ironically, the voice-over of symptoms helps sell drugs too. Some people listen carefully to the symptoms and then subconsciously repeat them later in the doctor's office. The ads sort of train them what to say to get the drug."

"Don't the ads make people fearful they might have a disease when they don't?"

"Sure. They make consumers feel that serious illness is

lurking around the corner. Ordinary heartburn becomes gas-troesophageal reflux disease. Occasional impotence caused by fatigue or alcohol becomes erectile dysfunction. The ads encourage people to make a decision to get a drug before hearing what their doctor has to say, basically diagnosing themselves. People who wouldn't touch the plumbing in their house, and aren't medically qualified, decide to take a drug they don't need based on a sixty-second TV commercial."

I knew the drug companies argue DTC ads make patients aware of important new treatments, and asked Barbara about that.

"Ads don't provide any useful overview of available treatments. They promote certain drugs only—generally costly new drugs for chronic conditions. Forty per cent of DTC spending in the U.S. is for just ten products. And few ads provide any evidence to support claims. They'll say something like 'clinically proven' or 'proven relief.' No one ever advertises older off-patent drugs, even if they are superior. DTC ads are not public health messages. They are promotions."

"They claim patients recognize their symptoms and avoid more serious disease by getting earlier treatment."

"Patients get information. But how accurate is it? One study identified more than half the drug ads in 1998 violated regulatory standards, usually exaggerating benefits and minimizing risks."[1]

"Prepulsid was promoted inappropriately. Do you know any other examples of where a drug promotion might have increased the number of people harmed by a risky drug?"

"Yes. A number of them. They advertised Rezulin in the U.S. for two years for diabetes after it was banned in the UK related to severe liver toxicity. The FDA asked them to withdraw it as the suspected cause of nearly four hundred deaths, sixty-three from liver failure."

That couldn't have happened if the warnings were clear, I thought. "In everything I've seen Big Pharma produce, the safety information is either missing, or buried in so much small print that it's virtually useless." Barbara agreed and concluded "With prescription drugs, safety information is not a frill. It's a crucial ingredient for maximizing benefit, and minimizing risk of prescription drugs. Without understanding both, drugs are worse than useless."

The night before my own testimony I stayed up very late going over my notes and research, preparing my words for the jury. Everything had come to this. I had no idea what conclusions the jury had drawn thus far, but I was very worried that some of the witnesses' thick resumés and the medical-speak had taken them off-track. The finger-pointing I'd seen in the last two weeks saddened me. Apparently no one did anything wrong; sometimes patients die out of the blue. These things happen. No one was to blame. Except the patient.

Day Sixteen
Monday, April 9, 2001

After fifteen days of witnesses and testimony, suddenly it was my turn. I'd condensed five lined pads of notes down to ten typed pages. Most important was filling in the blanks for the jury, where witnesses simply didn't know what Gloria and I knew. For example, the three doctors who had taken a history and spent time diagnosing Vanessa wrote in their files that despite a diagnosis of bulimia, she looked very healthy and her symptoms were under control. They were right. She was open and honest with the doctors about that, and had no electrolyte disorder. I had to tell the jury.

I had to correct misinformation the jury had heard through repeated questions. There was nothing wrong with

Vanessa's heart. The only time in her life she fainted she was on Prepulsid.

I also wanted to tell the jury what I had learned about the long history of Prepulsid and arrhythmias, and how the prescription drug industry operates. I wanted to explain "risk management," and about the published 1999 U.S. study that proved that doctors didn't read the Prepulsid label and warnings. Further deaths were inevitable. I would only have one chance to undo many days of blaming the victim, and try to undo the harm to Vanessa's reputation.

And I had assembled a list of thirty-nine recommendations for the jury from the Young family on how to make the drug surveillance system safer.

I remember vaguely when Gary Will called my name as a witness. My heart began to pound, and my face felt hot. This was it. Everyone was there because I had insisted on it. A lot of people were deeply involved in this "clean" death and counting on me. This had better be the presentation of my life. My testimony would be the key to keeping the oath I made to myself a year before—to expose the truth. Me and my ten pages of notes against these three formidable powers. All of a sudden I felt dreadfully inadequate.

As I walked to the stand, a dream I'd had the night before returned to me: a vivid memory of a summer night long ago, when Vanessa was two years old.

Vanessa had been crying after we put her down to bed. I went to her and she was standing in her crib with her pastel yellow Dr. Denton's sleeper on, her pretty face showing just above the rail. She was pointing at the window: "Monster," she whimpered. I heard nothing unusual, assumed she'd had a bad dream, and told her so. "It's OK Vanessa. Nothing's wrong. You can go to sleep." I went back downstairs.

A few minutes later little Vanessa was crying again—scared

by something. "What's wrong, Vanessa?" I asked. She pointed her tiny finger towards the window again—"Monster," she said, shaking her head up and down. "Vanessa, there are no monsters." I assured her. "That's just on TV." Puzzled, I listened. The only thing I heard was a noisy cricket down in the ravine. "Is that *noise* the monster?" I asked her. She shook her head yes. Mystery solved.

"Don't worry, Vanessa," I'd said. "That's just a little cricket, about this big." I spread my fingers and thumb an inch apart. "He couldn't hurt you. There are no such things as monsters. Tomorrow we'll go into the ravine and I'll show you what a little cricket looks like. OK?" She went right to sleep after that, trusting me. The next day we went into the ravine and I caught a cricket in my hand to show her. "See, Vanessa, no monster."

Vanessa studied the cricket in my hand. She was pleased. I'd kept my word. There were no monsters. She was safe. I took her little hand and we walked back to the house. It was strange. I could actually feel her hand.

I walked in front of the jury and turned around to occupy the stand. I took my own Bible out of my jacket pocket with my right hand—the one my godparents had given me when I was baptized at age one.

The coroner's clerk asked me to affirm my testimony. I said I would like to swear my testimony on the Bible my godparents had given me; the Bible I had taken to Vanessa's funeral; the Bible I would have one day taken to her wedding.

I swore on my Bible to tell the truth, and sat down. The dream wouldn't leave me. Gary Will was talking. I saw him and heard his voice in the distance. Everyone was looking at me. He was asking me a question.

I looked down at my notes and began to talk. I could hear my own voice. At first I responded to Gary Will's carefully planned questions. I spoke directly to the four jury members, looking each of them in the eye. Then I began to relate to the jury everything I'd learned over the last year.

I said it all. I held nothing back. First, I thanked everyone present for their efforts on behalf of Vanessa. Then I went to her defense. I told the jury if they took prescription drugs they were not safe. Vanessa's death was preventable, even predictable.

I explained how the lawyers had exaggerated Vanessa's problem to absolve everyone. Vanessa was a healthy girl whose one problem—throwing up—was under control. She weighed 137 pounds. I reminded them that the last doctor to see her said she was the picture of health. She slept well. She ate well. Out of three primary components of bulimia—binge eating, laxatives (diuretics), and throwing up—she only had one, throwing up. She was not a binge eater and never used diuretics or laxatives. They weren't allowed in our house. I told them how she occasionally had headaches and might have suffered what is called "abdominal migraine." Records showed she had no sign of an electrolyte disorder, lots of energy, and a "peaches and cream" complexion. I gave them the important missing detail about the psychiatrist's clinic and how Vanessa had felt humiliated by the reception she and Gloria had received. And I made it clear that Gloria and Vanessa did not forget, or in any way mislead her or her occupational therapist, that Vanessa sometimes took Prepulsid, but filled out a badly worded form correctly.

I related how her psychiatrist was cheerful and made Vanessa laugh, building almost instant rapport. I explained risk management, and that because Health Canada was Big Pharma's key customer, instead of ordering dangerous drugs off the market Health Canada negotiates with the drug companies, wasting precious time and extending risks to patients.

Frankly, I was afraid I would be cut off. The coroner could do so at any time. But he never did. He'd ruled out some crucial written documents—like the exposé from the *L.A. Times*, because this was an inquest, not a trial. But for the same reason I was given a lot of latitude in my testimony. He honoured my one chance to speak out.

And the lawyers for the other side didn't object. I assume they didn't want to make the jury any more sympathetic to me than I would otherwise be. I have to admit if I was a lawyer for the doctors or Johnson & Johnson I would have objected.

Referring to my own background in marketing and communications, I outlined how easily effective warnings about Prepulsid could have been issued by Health Canada: a clearly worded "Dear Doctor" letter in a brightly coloured envelope sent out within forty-eight hours (as they did with AZT), a press conference, full-page ads in the newspapers, a request for the Minister of Health—who was ultimately responsible—to get involved. I told them bluntly if our regulator or Johnson & Johnson had done any of the above Vanessa would be alive.

I can't remember everything I said. But I think I also reiterated how our doctor knew Vanessa might be taking 50 mg a day of Prepulsid—10 mgs over the maximum daily adult dose and said nothing. And I reminded them how Johnson & Johnson had issued the highest level of warning—a black box warning in the U.S. in 1998 and done nothing similar in Canada. Public Citizen, who received no government or pharma money, had told *Worst Pills–Best Pills* readers "Do not take" Prepulsid back in 1999, because the risks did not exceed the benefits.

I pointed out that Wendy Arnott had testified that safety was Janssen-Ortho's most important priority, yet before February 2000 not one of Vanessa's doctors knew the true risks of Prepulsid, a complete failure on that priority.

I described how every time Johnson & Johnson had revised the Prepulsid label to add new dangers, it turned out to be incomplete and new dangers appeared. So what's to say the current label used in other countries today is complete?

I reiterated that Wendy Arnott had testified repeatedly that their detail reps were out to promote safe use of Prepulsid, yet not one healthcare professional who appeared at this inquest testified they'd ever heard a word about the risks from any of them.

I advised them there were a number people in positions of power who with one simple act in the interest of patient safety could have saved Vanessa's life.

I talked for a long time. Well over an hour. I outlined thirty-nine recommendations to the jury to prevent further similar deaths. Things like an independent drug safety agency, compulsory adverse reaction reporting for doctors, clearly worded warnings to be handed to patients with every prescription. All the suggestions I'd heard from experts in the last year.

The jury listened attentively. They seemed to be very interested.

It was over before I knew it. I prayed I had been convincing.

The next day, Wednesday, the parties made final submissions to the jury, and on Thursday the coroner gave his directions to the jury. It was over. Except for the jury's decision.

They'd heard sixteen days of testimony and by law had three primary tasks. The first was to determine by what means Vanessa died: homicide, suicide, natural, or accidental. To help us, it had to be accidental. Because in Ontario, "natural" includes medical error. If the jury decided the means of death was natural, Prepulsid was off the hook.

Their second duty was to determine the cause of death. There was no issue that Vanessa died due to a heart arrhythmia. But everything depended on the jury saying Prepulsid was the cause, or at least one of the causes, of that arrhythmia. If the jury somehow came to the conclusion that Dr. George Klein was right, and Vanessa just died out of the blue as a complete coincidence, it would be a huge setback, maybe the end for our civil case. Could I expect Gary Will to fight a civil case for five years that appeared to have little chance of succeeding?

The third duty was to make recommendations to the government for changes to the system to prevent similar deaths in the future. I hoped they would accept my suggestions. My life would be on hold until the jury's verdict—expected in a few weeks.

I WAS STILL TRYING TO GET THE STORY out about the seven out of ten deaths at Joseph Brant Hospital in Burlington. Gary had asked the Health Canada doctor about it on the stand. He'd described the report as a cluster of ten deaths that came from one individual, submitted with very little information, who refused to provide them with any further information. I know Sana had sent them the further information they asked for. The *Burlington Post* covered the story, and the *Globe and Mail* did a brief story, but the other major newspapers seemed disinterested. At first I couldn't figure out why.

Barbara Mintzes had not been critical of the role of the media in DTC advertising. But I began to see potential conflicts of interest. Based on my political experience, I doubted that the drug companies would spend huge amounts of money on ads in newspapers or on TV stations that went out of their way to cover stories that hurt their industry. In fact the stories on adverse drug reactions that did appear were usually after patients had died, stories that virtually had to be reported. And new drugs, or drugs still in development, were usually described strictly in glowing terms.

In my research I discovered I wasn't alone in my cynicism. In 1999, 78 per cent of Americans told the American Society of Newspaper Editors that "powerful people can get stories into the paper or keep them out."[2] By April 2003, the Canadian

Centre for Policy Alternatives reported that Canada's largest twenty-four daily newspapers gave Canadians incomplete information on five major new prescription drugs, promoting unrealistic expectations about their benefits, usually describing them in terms like "highly effective" or "proven remedy," right out of the press releases.[3] And a lot of important information was missing. Only one out of three of the stories even mentioned possible adverse effects, which were usually downplayed using terms like "minor" or "rare." Contraindications were only mentioned in 4 per cent of the articles.

To be blunt, in keeping patients safe, the media is part of the solution, but also part of the problem.

Relative Benefit vs. Absolute Benefit
How 1 per cent becomes 50 per cent

Four out of five U.S. news stories report the "relative" benefit of the drugs.[4] Basically that's how bullshit baffles brains. For example, many 1996 stories claimed that Fosamax would cut female patients' risk of hip fractures in half. Doesn't that sound amazing? Half! Who *wouldn't* consider taking a drug that helpful? But hold on: the true risk of having a broken hip for elderly women over a period of time is about 2 per cent. That's two out of one hundred women over many years. The stories claimed a 50 per cent reduction in relative risk for Fosamax. Relative to what? Relative to those who broke a hip. So the best result Fosamax could truly claim was a reduction in risk from 2 in 100 women, to 1 in 100 women. For a large group of women taking Fosamax for years, one woman would break her hip, not two. Maybe. That's called 1 per cent "absolute" reduction risk. Not quite as amazing is it?[5]

And Fosamax can have some nasty side effects. Rotting (necrosis) of the jaw has shown up as a rare side effect. And a recent study appears to show that long-term use makes bones more brittle, so they might break more easily.[6] Maybe after more research, that 1 per cent absolute benefit will be cancelled out by a 1 per cent rate of adverse effects. That's a lot different than reducing risk by "half" when we started, isn't it?

Why aren't the news media editors challenging the marketing hype? One possibility is that Big Pharma spends over $4 billion a year in the U.S. on DTC ads, and the media gets the money. I don't believe direct deals are made to leave out news, or that our media refuse to tell us bad news about Big Pharma. Some stories are certainly covered. I've quoted a lot of them. But it never ceases to amaze me how little the average person knows about the risks of taking prescription drugs. Full-page ads purchased by drug companies—at cost of $20,000 to $65,000 each—can make a significant difference on the bottom line of a newspaper or magazine. And when advertisers just stop calling, someone must start asking questions. Four hundred million dollars a year in drug money is currently on the table in Canada for our media if the courts allow open DTC advertising here.[7] Four hundred million dollars could buy a lot of silence.

In the months after losing Vanessa, Gloria and I found refuge in watching comedy reruns on TV. One evening one of them was interrupted by the site of a middle-aged man's body being slowly pulled out in a morgue drawer. Next we saw the man's wife and children weeping hopelessly, and then what we assumed was the same man at a family picnic falling down, obviously in great pain. Shock, sadness, and fear all in the middle of a favourite TV show. A haunting voice in the background was telling us who was at risk of this fate: women fifty years or older; men forty years or older; anyone who is overweight, physically inactive, a smoker or has high blood pressure, has heart disease, diabetes, or family history of heart disease or high cholesterol. In other words, probably more than half the population. For those who don't watch TV, the full-page "toe tag" ad—showing the feet of a body with a toe tag—appeared in our newspapers and magazines for months under the headline: "Which would you rather have, a cholesterol test or a final exam?"

Take a test or die.

Of course they omit a third choice—ignore fear-mongering ads. This ad campaign was very successful. But Health Canada officials claimed the toe tag campaign was a help-seeking ad and was not advertising. The ads displayed the logos of the Canadian Diabetes Association and Canadian Lipid Nurse Network, and in tiny print at the very bottom of the page these words: "Sponsored by one of Canada's research-based pharmaceutical companies."[8] The name Pfizer does not appear because it's not technically supposed to be an ad for a drug. But Pfizer money was behind the toe tag campaign to sell more Lipitor—the world's biggest-selling drug at over $14 billion a year. And you can bet any ad that looks like a public service announcement sending you to "ask your doctor" is also a drug ad. To my eyes Pfizer used the Canadian Diabetes Association and the Lipid Nurse Network to make the ad appear to be a public service message, and lower people's commercial guard.[9]

Why would Pfizer spend millions of dollars on ads that don't name the product or their company? Because they have an ace in the hole—our doctors—who will.

Most patients believe drug ads,[10] and the ads herd patients into doctor's offices, where they get the drugs. In one study three out of four actresses requesting a drug on unscheduled visits to doctors' offices were given a prescription upon request. A U.S. Consumers Reports study showed that *two out of three doctors* will give a patient a drug they request at least some of the time, but advised their readers to ignore drug ads.[11]

My question is: are these doctors or order-takers? Why

would doctors write out scrips seemingly on request? One reason I found out is repeat business. In one study 28 per cent of patients said they would switch doctors to get a desired medicine.[12] Big Pharma would not be surprised. They track every doctor by prescription and their $4 billion investment on DTC ads pays off, big time. Americans now see an average of over ten drug ads every day.[13] That's why drug costs in the U.S. continue to climb far beyond the rate of inflation every year, along with DTC spending.[14]

Drug ads raise our emotions, like fear: a woman walking on a blurred and crowded city street for Paxil; or embarrassment: a man abandoning a business meeting to go to the washroom for Avodart.[15] When we are emotional it's hard to think. Big Pharma wants you to make an emotional decision to get a drug, and your beleaguered doctor has to try to talk you out of it. The danger is that drug ads exaggerate effectiveness and downplay risks. Drugs aren't shampoo or hand lotion. False promises about drugs could end up getting you hurt. In November 2005 a poll reported in the *New York Times* showed that only 9 per cent of Americans believed that drug companies are generally honest. Could that be one reason why?

Chapter 20

The Butterfly Effect

"So long as little children are allowed to suffer, there is no love in this world."
—Isodora Duncan

GARY WILL CALLED ME on Thursday, April 19, 2001: "The jury will report its verdict to the coroner next Tuesday. Can you be there?" There was no question I would be.

Once again that Tuesday I drove alongside the transport trailers on the QEW to Hamilton, waited to get through the metal detectors at the John Sopinka Courthouse, and sat in the front row of Courtroom 600. It seemed like months ago that I'd been there. I knew that day would forever change my life, sending me along a new road, whatever the jury's decision. I was profoundly afraid that Vanessa's short life would be discarded by our legal system.

I tried to make eye contact with the jury members as they came in their private door, but none of them looked my way. Not good, I thought. These four people held my fate in their hands and I knew nothing about them except their names: Kerry

Bruder, Michelle Fraser, Sharon Jamieson, and Craig Wolf. I truly didn't know which way their decision would go. Everyone stood as the coroner entered and sat down. Having received the jury's report, the coroner prepared to read their verdict out loud.

The first decision to be announced was the means of death. The jury would certainly not choose murder or suicide. "Natural causes" meant by "natural disease process" but could include medical error. If the jury chose natural causes it was over. It had to be "accidental."

There was total silence in the courtroom. Then the coroner spoke:

"The jury finds the means of death was accidental." Thank God.

Next he would announce the cause of death. I stopped breathing and literally closed my eyes.

"Acute hypoxic/ischemic encephalopathy due to cardiac arrhythmia by cardiac arrest ..."

That was OK. We knew that.

"... resulting from the effects of bulimia nervosa ..."

I expected that.

"... in conjunction with cisapride toxicity ..." I opened my eyes, and ran the words through my mind repeatedly: cisapride toxicity.

There it was. Mercy for Vanessa. Hope for our case. I exhaled. Cisapride had poisoned Vanessa. The world would know.

"... and possibly an unknown co-factor such as a congenital cardiac defect ..."

Professor George Klein had persuaded the jury—just a little.

I will never know if having four jurors instead of five made any difference, but at least two of them must have been swayed enough to insist the decision include the *possibility* of an unknown co-factor. Now I could see how so few drugs are exposed as dangerous in our courts. If the drug companies could use expert witnesses to subtly persuade juries to abandon "on the balance of probabilities"—what was probable—and think "cause and effect," it was almost impossible for plaintiffs to prove a drug caused an adverse reaction death. All the companies had to do was convince a jury that anybody could die at any time, without warning—from a previously undiagnosed conduction defect—and they might walk away. The best part of Dr. Klein's theory for Big Pharma was there didn't have to be any evidence.

But it didn't matter today. By the standard in this inquest cisapride was the poison. It was a cause of death. The jury had been wise.

Gary Will had done a superb job. The opposition had failed to have Vanessa blamed for her own death. Before I knew it, the coroner had thanked the jury and excused them. The lawyers were still talking at the front of the courtroom but I couldn't hear them. My mind was racing. I was experiencing grief and a kind of elation at the same time.

The network TV cameras and Erna Buffie's film crew were waiting across the street in Courthouse Square. Gary and I went down in the elevator for the last time, went through the lobby, and crossed the street. We watched and listened in silence as Wendy Arnott, vice-president at Janssen-Ortho gave her prepared statement, saying in part: "Prepulsid is safe and effective when used according to the prescribing information." The Big Pharma mantra. With five new labels over seven years and new contraindications almost every year, that had never been true. And it was highly unlikely it was true that day either. But they were still selling the stuff in many countries so it was still all about the mantra—and sales.

Then in response to a question, Wendy Arnott made an on-camera comment I will never forget: she referred to Vanessa as an "inappropriate candidate" for Prepulsid. As far as Janssen-Ortho was concerned nothing had changed. The drug was fine;

just some of the patients were a problem. She made it sound like Vanessa had been turned down for a job instead of dying.

In August Ms. Arnott sent a letter to the *Canadian Medical Association Journal* denying that cisapride caused Vanessa's death, saying Vanessa had "risk factors for cardiac rhythm problems that could have caused her death independently of any medication she may have been taking." The jury never said that. They said "possibly an unknown co-factor." When I saw this letter I was reminded of testimony Ms. Arnott gave at the inquest. Gary Will had asked if the sales data Janssen-Ortho purchased from IMS was used by their sales force to encourage doctors to prescribe more Prepulsid. She said, "No, again I think the role of our sales force is not necessarily to encourage more prescriptions." And she looked quite serious.

Vanessa was gone. But our case, and my goals were alive. In Hamilton, Ontario, the first Prepulsid jury case in North America out of the chute was a bad omen for Johnson & Johnson.

The jury also made fifty-nine recommendations for improving drug safety in Canada directed at Health Canada, the pharmaceutical industry, the Ontario College of Physicians and Surgeons, the Ontario College of Pharmacists, the Ontario College of Family Physicians, Ontario Medical Schools, the Ontario College of Nurses, the Ontario Ministry of Health, and the Ontario Coroner's Office which included:

- Health Canada should mandate drug companies to clearly indicate important safety information on labels, prescribing information, and promotional material
- mandatory reporting of all serious adverse drug reactions within 48 hours for healthcare professionals
- Dear Doctor letters should be clearly marked, approved, and issued by Health Canada, not the drug companies

- Drug companies should provide safety messages for new risk information on detail rep visits to doctors, on information phone lines, and even websites
- Health Canada should develop a "template" for patient information leaflets that is "clear, concise, and easily understood"
- Drug companies should ensure broad media coverage of important warning information (like press releases and visible alerts in newspapers)
- Drug companies should ensure that adverse reaction information be as effectively communicated to doctors as initial marketing information

There was a lot more—such as a monthly bulletin of drug news, a global database of ADR reports, and a legal requirement for drug companies to report any label changes or rejection of their drugs for specific indications in foreign countries. The jury had agreed with many of my recommendations and even went much further. Their report, if implemented, would revolutionize drug safety in Canada and save thousands of lives.

Under the law, Health Canada had a year to report back to the coroner about what they had done. Unfortunately, these were non-binding recommendations.

There was no celebration at the Young household that evening, only a tremendous sense of relief. I really felt like we had been blessed. Gloria had heard the result on the radio before I got home. I called Madeline in Kingston to tell her that Prepulsid was named as a primary cause of death, and told Hart when he came in from school. Each of us had a private place in our heart for times like this. One step, one day at a time. We all knew it would be years before we had any closure.

I renewed my research the next day. The next challenge was our lawsuit. And in a civil trial the rules would be different. It was highly unlikely the judge would rule my binder of published studies, and David Willman's *L.A. Times* exposé as irrelevant. On the other hand, neither would a trial judge allow me to say many of the things I'd said at the inquest on the stand. We served the class action on Johnson & Johnson and Health Canada a week later.

I continued to follow the litigation in the U.S. carefully. About 16,000 U.S. Prepulsid plaintiffs, including three hundred death claims, were assembled into one Multi-District Litigation out of New Orleans. The case never went to trial. What happened in February 2004 was strikingly similar to the story in John Grisham's novel *King of Torts*. The lawyers would divide up as much as $22.5 million, and an administration fee of $15 million was established. The plaintiffs would divide up to $90 million. Each plaintiff would appear before a mediator and plead their case for damages. What did Johnson & Johnson get in exchange? Over one million documents sealed forever, that showed . . . what? What kind of information could have been worth over $90 million to seal up, without defending Prepulsid in open court? I knew exactly what kind of information that was sealed. And I think you do as well. It was the kind of information that could be worth hundreds of millions of dollars in damages if the majority of the claimants insisted on a trial.

By 2006 Merck faced over $20 billion in lawsuits for Vioxx. That, also is risk management. I admit I tried for months to get those sealed Prepulsid documents from allies in the U.S. As I don't live under U.S. law I was not restricted from seeing them. I asked many of my U.S. contacts if they were available. But if they had them, no one would give them to me.

In the meanwhile the lawyers for Johnson & Johnson had been arguing their position against our class action being certified in an Ontario court. In the ensuing years they brought six motions to court on various legal points, each like a small trial in itself, requiring legal arguments and a written judicial decision.

In May of 2005 we were simply not much further ahead. We were past "deny" but stuck in "delay."

June 11, 2005

As usual, first thing that morning I went down to my home office, now in the finished basement of a new house we'd bought in the same neighbourhood in 2002. I set down my cup of tea, clicked with my mouse on an email title that had caught my attention, and sat in stunned silence. There it was. The *New York Times* had done a startling exposé on Prepulsid: "Lucrative Drug, Danger Signals and the F.D.A."[1] I sat in silent comprehension staring at my screen reading, my heart pounding.

I read it three times. "This will change everything," I said quietly to myself.

The picture it painted was not pretty. This was the first published evidence I had seen that Johnson & Johnson withheld safety information to keep sales up. Janssen had fought the FDA on the wording of a safety warning on the Prepulsid label *because they felt it might cost $250 million in lost sales.* The fact that Janssen managers had even calculated what the warning on the label would cost in lost sales sickened me. Human life on the same continuum as profits.

Reports had mounted since way back in 1993 about drug-induced serious heart arrhythmias and "a growing number of cardiac problems in infants and children" leading the FDA to suggest "that pediatric patients may be at greater risk." Johnson & Johnson didn't conduct safety studies the FDA had recommended.

Instead of sending out truly effective warnings about off-label pediatric use, in the U.S. Johnson & Johnson continued to underwrite efforts to promote its use in babies who spat up. Instead of taking the drug off the market, Johnson & Johnson hired Dr. Paul Hyman, a pediatric gastroenterologist, to convince other physicians that Prepulsid was safe for children. He made presentations to thousands of doctors.

At a March 1998 meeting with Johnson & Johnson officials, a slide projected by an FDA official read, "Is it acceptable for your nighttime heartburn medicine (i.e., something for which you could take Tums) to have the potential to kill you?"

And Johnson & Johnson never proved Prepulsid even worked for children! A secret internal memo written by Dr. Janice Bush, VP of Global Regulatory Affairs at Janssen Research Foundation, just weeks before Vanessa died, said, "Do we want to stand in front of the world and admit we were never able to prove efficacy?" She had underlined the words "never able."[2]

My memory of that summer night long ago flashed through my mind. "There's no such thing as monsters, Vanessa," I'd said. And she'd trusted me.

My mind was racing. Our battle could be over. This must be the information I'd been trying to obtain. A U.S. court had ordered it sealed, but journalists Gardiner Harris and Eric Koli had unearthed it. I couldn't imagine Janssen executives successfully defending this story before a jury in a civil trial. Even if they tried, no one at Johnson & Johnson would want these facts paraded in front of a Canadian jury and journalists day after day, fodder for the nightly news and national papers. Someone had sent me a wonderful gift. It felt like Christmas morning. I forwarded the article to Gary Will with a note: "Gary this is what I've been looking for!" What an understatement. I went upstairs and told Gloria that the tables had turned. It was hard to believe that one newspaper story could make such a huge difference in our lives. But I felt it would.

Sana Sukkari never backed down. Heroes rarely do. She and Larry Sasich from Public Citizen got married, and she continued to stand up for her patients at Joseph Brant Hospital until February 28, 2006, when she and the hospital parted ways. She never felt those around her there had the knowledge or the will to understand her commitment to patient safety. The coroner who investigated the deaths at Joseph Brant Hospital related to Prepulsid—Dr. Karen Acheson—unsurprisingly found no "cause and effect" in the seven Prepulsid-related deaths, and in her one-page report never even mentioned the fact that seven out of ten patients were given Prepulsid when it was contraindicated. Other than Sana, Larry, and the drug safety advocates I'd met, no one seemed to care. Sana is now an assistant professor at LECOM School of Pharmacy, the same school as Larry in Erie, Pennsylvania.

Gloria left work and began taking cooking courses part-time at George Brown College. She now has her chef's diploma. Madeline got her B.A. from Queen's and a diploma in directing opera through Massey College at University of Toronto. Hart switched high schools in grade ten, and again in grade twelve to Abbey Park High School where he graduated with honours. He's currently studying Landscape Architecture at Guelph University. I continue my advocacy through Drug Safety Canada, which I founded in 2002.

I ran as the Conservative candidate for Oakville in the 2006 federal election, coming within 744 votes of unseating the incumbent, and again on October 14, 2008, this time winning the riding. As MP for Oakville, I will be an additional voice in Ottawa for improved regulations, especially the need for truly effective safety warnings given to patients with their prescription. And I will work to break up the inappropriate Big Pharma "partnerships" with our doctors and regulators that is so unhealthy for patients.

I was never able to prove my molecular theory—that cisapride, bepridil, astemizole and the other Johnson & Johnson drugs that caused long QT might have come from one original molecule, and that's why they all caused heart arrhythmias.

Someone else will have to take that on. Dr. Paul Janssen died in 2003 and these are trade secrets, so we might never know.

Producer Erna Buffie and Director Elise Swerhone's excellent short film *Drug Deals: The Brave New World of Prescription Drugs*, was produced for the National Film Board and broadcast on CBC's *The Nature of Things* in November 2001. It won two awards.[3]

Gary Will won his appeal to the Supreme Court of Canada—the Pilot Insurance Case—on February 22, 2002. Canadian Supreme Court Justice William Binnie restored the jury award of punitive damages of $1 million. It stands as a landmark in Canadian law for plaintiffs.

On January 11, 2006, Gardiner Harris at the *New York Times* was stirring up bad PR for the drug industry again. Actually it was the U.S. Congress Senate Finance Committee, who reported that twenty-three pharma companies had spent $1.47 billion on "educational grants" for doctors in 2004. The committee letter that was sent to Johnson & Johnson mentioned that Johnson & Johnson had provided more than $1.3 million to one patient group. The *Times* concluded that this could be the same group that had made thousands of presentations on treating childhood reflux to pediatric doctors and nurses recommending Prepulsid. The group folded after Prepulsid was pulled off the market in 2000.

In the meanwhile Johnson & Johnson had been awarded the 2003 Most Caring Corporation in America Award by The Caring Institute, of Washington D.C., a group inspired by the inspiration of Mother Theresa, and chaired by former Viagra spokesman Robert Dole. According to the Caring Institute website, regarding Johnson & Johnson, by "SEC and company records there is only one product liability case pending, involving a drug 'Prepulsid' made by their Janssen Pharmaceutical Subsidiary. A judgment of $48 million against the company is being appealed, based on facts elicited at the trial that no one bringing the lawsuit was injured by taking the drug."

On January 18, 2007—over six years after I filed the Canadian Prepulsid class action, and after our lawyers fought six motions by Johnson & Johnson—Madame Justice Ellen M. MacDonald of the Ontario Superior Court of Justice certified the action to go ahead. Johnson & Johnson also appealed the certification, but lost that appeal in May 2007. They appealed that decision and lost as well. As of September 2007 the Canadian class action for Prepulsid was finally moving ahead in Ontario. Vanessa would have been twenty-four.

I suspect in time Johnson & Johnson will settle with the Canadian plaintiffs. The last thing they want is the information from the *New York Times* exposé and this book splashed on the front pages of our newspapers and in the worldwide media again, where it might get the attention of another parent who has lost a child in India, or Taiwan, where cisapride is still prescribed for children with other drugs, even though it was banned by the Taiwan Department of Health in 2005 after two deaths.[4]

Someone stubborn like me.

It took until February 2006, but we finally settled our individual lawsuit against Johnson & Johnson—out of court. Our decision to settle was determined by the state of Canadian law, which we found makes justice almost inaccessible for plaintiffs in such cases. There is no balance of power between powerless individuals and huge international corporations as there is in the U.S. There was nothing I wanted more than a public trial exposing all the things I've told you in this book. But if I had insisted on our day in court by refusing to settle at a mediation, I was taking a terrible risk of having to pay the legal costs of the defendants, possibly over $1 million, and losing our home. It was unthinkable. My family had suffered too much already. It was clearly time to give up my legal battle.

But I agonized that in doing so I was abandoning Vanessa, betraying the oath I made in her name the morning after she died. With the help of friends and family I concluded that although no jury would ever expose who was responsible for Vanessa's death, this book would get the story out. That would fulfill my oath to expose the truth. I am very grateful to Key Porter for taking a chance on me.

In February 2006, Gloria, Madeline, and I joined Gary Will at 10 a.m. in a mediation centre on the top floor of First Canadian Place. Hart was in London, Ontario, at Fanshawe College. Former Supreme Court Justice Peter Cory acted as mediator, and at 10:15 that evening the parties came to a settlement in our individual case. As part of that agreement, I am only allowed to say is that the case was settled to the satisfaction of all parties.

I keep my word.

Epilogue

Who Killed Vanessa?

WAS VANESSA'S DEATH IN VAIN? On that question, the jury is still out. Between the time Prepulsid was ordered off the Canadian market in August 2000, having been made available by special access only, and May 2007, it has been reported to Health Canada as suspected in forty-five adverse reactions, including the death of a seven-month-old male infant taking no other drugs.[1] It's difficult to estimate the true number of serious reactions for a drug available only by special access, but it would be naive to think Health Canada got reports on them all.

Has Health Canada sharpened up their operation?

In July 2007 they listed cisapride and Prepulsid under different headings on their ADR database, as if they were different active ingredients. If patients or doctors didn't think to check both names and add them up, they'd be misled about the number of reactions caused by Prepulsid. They did the same with Zyban, Wellbutrin, and buprophion, which also all have the exact same active ingredient: an antidepressant. I spoke to Health Canada officials on a conference call to suggest they combine them on the same list. "That's a good idea," they said. By September the drugs were still listed separately.

What about the jury's fifty-nine recommendations?

As president of Drug Safety Canada, I am sorry to tell you that prescription drugs are still killing our loved ones, perhaps at the same or higher rate. Drug labels and warnings are still confusing. No clearly worded comprehensive Medguides are given out with prescriptions like they are in the U.S.

And the call I made for an independent drug agency for Canada—although supported by the Romanow Commission in 2003—is still a dream.

Since 2003 Health Canada officials have been proposing to modernize the Food and Drugs Act, developing a concept called "progressive licensing," intended, according to their website, "to give Canadians a regulatory system that supports access to the drugs that will help them maintain and improve their health." They had proposed a pre-submission body for determining which drugs would qualify for a *departure* from traditional standards. Did they mean the standards were too high? Or too low?

However, by April 2008 the minister of health, the Honourable Tony Clement, introduced significant changes to the Food and Drugs Act, as part of the Food and Consumer Safety Action Plan, including a commitment to develop regulations for mandatory adverse drug reaction reporting from hospitals, to empower Health Canada officials to order drug recalls directly, and to coerce manufacturers to demonstrate that drugs already on the market continue to remain safe and effective. These are all very positive steps.

Companies could also be required to provide information on authorized clinical trials, and compile and report information on any therapeutic product to the minister. The minister may also order revisions to a drug label to prevent injury to health. These changes could help put an end to the drawn-out negotiations between Health Canada and pharmaceutical-company linguists over the fine print on drug labels while Canadians are dying.

However, the Big Pharma companies (by way of their lobby group Rx&D) appear to be unfussed about these changes, so drug safety advocates are asking: is "progressive licensing" just Health Canada pharma-speak for determining how safe drugs are *after* we and our family members take them—the dreaded risk management? They are wondering if the bureaucrats at Health Canada have made some sort of side deal with their partners in health care—verbal commitments that under the changes new drug applications will be processed faster, a dangerous practice. When I was MPP, I had witnessed a disturbing operational assumption amongst senior bureaucrats: "governments may come and go, but we will always be here."

This story is far from over.

The safe use of prescription drugs holds the highest potential to save lives and reduce injury in our hands today. We don't need any miraculous discoveries. We don't need to invest billions in technology or new treatments. In fact our governments would *save* billions of dollars currently spent on inappropriate prescription drug use, and medical care for hundreds of thousands of adverse drug reaction victims. But humanity is the key. We just have to find ways to ensure patients only use prescription drugs when they are safe—get back to the precautionary principle.

It's not just integrity that the drug industry, the medical profession, and our regulatory system needs. It's truly putting patients first—mercy.

Who killed Vanessa? When it was all said and done, I think the ultimate enemy was self-interest. Professional people in positions of trust neglected to do what they knew they should have. Others, concerned about their jobs and careers, turned a blind eye to dangers to which they would never have exposed their own families. They turned off their sense of right and wrong when they went to work each day.

But the people who casually manipulated the self-interest of others, and acted to delay and undermine effective warnings that would have saved Vanessa's life deserve special recognition. Perhaps I was wrong when I promised Vanessa there was no such thing as monsters. They don't look like the ones children see on television or movies, or hide in dark ravines making scary noises. They look like everyone else, and live in beautiful homes. They are the monsters we should all be afraid of. By now you know who they are.

No doubt, one day our children's children will learn in school that in the early part of the twenty-first century tens of thousands of people died every year after taking unnecessary drugs that did little for their health. They'll learn that there were no effective laws to protect people from risky drugs. It is my hope this book helps to make the changes we need to end this era.

Sometimes when I worked alone at night at my desk I wondered what God would do with a beautiful human spirit like Vanessa. She loved babies, especially our neighbours David and Ann's little girl who she babysat, calling her "my baby." In my hundreds of hours of research, the stories that chilled me were when children suffered after being given experimental drugs. One particular story from 1996 stayed with me.[2] A ten-year-old girl in Nigeria who had contracted meningitis in an outbreak had died *along with ninety-nine others* after being given the experimental drug Trovan for three days, and no other antibiotic.[3]

There were no records that the children given Trovan or that their parents understood they were part of an experiment, and she was identified only as Patient No. 0069.

I began to wonder, who greets children when they get to heaven before their parents? Wouldn't ten-year-old Patient No. 0069 from Nigeria feel disoriented and confused at her own passing to the afterlife? She would need a friendly face and someone to take her hand to show her around. It would have to be someone like Vanessa. She would have no doubt she was meeting an angel.

Afterword

Sunday May 7, 2007

WE'D BEEN IN A NEW HOUSE for five years, and the legal settlement for our lawsuit was completed the year before. Hart was twenty, and having completed his second year at Fanshawe College in London had moved back into his loft in our Oakville house while working for the summer. Madeline has just completed her studies in directing opera through Massey College at University of Toronto. Life was in many ways getting back to normal. Which is why it was so distressing when tragedy struck in our community again.

The phone rang at 9 p.m. Hart answered and listened briefly, said a few words and then hung up. He was visibly distraught. "Sara Carlin hung herself," he managed to say. Sara was a beautiful, vibrant eighteen-year-old Oakville girl, part of Hart's group of friends who loved to hang out and party, gathering for Karaoke night at local night spots. Sara had been at our house a few weeks before.

And now she was gone. My first thought was about her family—the dread of what they were about to go through. But my second was suspicion. Sara had apparently hung herself in the basement of her home some time on Saturday night. Her father found her fully suspended at 4:30 p.m. on Sunday. I could only imagine his horror. But a young woman hanging herself like that is an extremely rare occurrence.

Sara had been a high achiever at school, in sports, music, and at her part-time job, until early 2006 when she had been prescribed an SSRI antidepressant—GlaxoSmithKline block-buster Paxil—for anxiety.[1] Then her behaviour began to change. She quit her high school hockey team and her part-time job at an optometrist's office. She began to suffer from insomnia and her behaviour deteriorated as she got involved with recreational drugs and began to abuse alcohol. Sara's father, Neil, described her as a completely different person.

Tragically, no one had told Sara or her family that Health Canada had already issued two Dear Healthcare Professional letters about Paxil and suicide. The first, in July 2003, said Paxil should not be prescribed to anyone under eighteen years old because it could increase their risk of suicide. It also cautioned against the abrupt discontinuation of the drug, because that might cause "discontinuation symptoms," one of them referred to in medical-speak as "suicide-related adverse events." Sara had abruptly stopped taking Paxil several days before she died, and then started taking it again, by the record taking six pills over thirty-six hours, perhaps in an attempt to catch up. Paxil users are most likely to suffer adverse effects when the dosage changes up or down, like getting on or off a moving train.

The second Health Canada letter in May 2004 issued a stronger warning to physicians for Paxil regarding the risk of self-harm and behavioural and emotional changes, including agitation, hostility, disinhibition, depersonalization, and akathesia. Akathesia has been described as an extreme inner restlessness accompanied by overwhelming anxiety, malaise, and even severe dysphoria *manifesting as an almost indescribable sense of terror and doom.*

For some patients Paxil could be a kind of torture.

The *Canadian Medical Association Journal* had reported just two months before that 10.5 per cent of pediatric and adolescent patients on Paxil dropped out of clinical trials because of serious psychiatric events like "emotional lability" which includes suicidal ideation, conduct problems, hostility, and "abnormal thinking," which might include two additional problems Sara had never before experienced: alcohol abuse, which was also observed during Paxil trials, and the use of illicit substances.[2]

Sara's death was déjà vu for me. Five "Dear Doctor" warning letters had gone out from Health Canada about Paxil—just like Prepulsid. And neither Sara nor her family had been told about any of them.[3] Nor had they been told that GlaxoSmith-Kline had been under criminal investigation for three years in the UK regarding Paxil (named Seroxat there) or that GSK had paid $2.5 million to help settle a 2004 lawsuit initiated by the state of New York alleging that they engaged in repeated and persistent fraud by concealing and failing to disclose information concerning Paxil's safety and efficacy for children and teens.

Paxil had also, like Prepulsid five years before, been the subject of an article in the *Canadian Adverse Reaction Newsletter* in 2003 because doctors could not tell if it was safe.[4]

Those were the conditions under which Sara Carlin's doctor had given her Paxil.

It gets worse. In January 2008, the *New England Journal of Medicine* reported that publication bias in Medical Journals had totally skewed doctor's conclusions about the effectiveness of SSRI antidepressants.[5] In March 2008 British reports were published showing SSRI antidepressants—including Paxil—"generally worked no better that dummy pills."[6]

By this time I'd learned that both shooters at the Columbine massacre in Littleton, Colorado, had been on SSRI antidepressants and researched these drugs at length. In almost every other case I could find where someone had taken a gun to school and started shooting there were credible reports the shooters were on, or withdrawing from, an antidepressant.

SSRIstories.com catalogues over 2,400 acts of bizarre behaviour, mostly criminal, committed by patients on blockbuster antidepressants including self-mutilation, attempted suicide, suicide, homicide, multiple homicide, robbery, road rage, arson, and school shootings.[7]

The amazing thing to me was that suicidal ideation and sometimes even homicidal ideation—wanting to kill someone— are printed as possible side effects right on the labels of these drugs. Yet physicians prescribe them widely for common anxiety due to social pressures or exams, and even mild depression that would get better over time.[8]

SSRI drug labels tell doctors that patients taking these drugs should be closely monitored. By whom? I wonder. The U.S. Paxil label says: "Families and caregivers of patients should be advised to look for the emergence of such symptoms on a day-to-day basis, since changes may be abrupt." It sounds like Paxil is not safe unless the patient's family, spouse, or roommate commit themselves to participate in a daily suicide watch. Yet no one had said a word about suicide risk to Sara Carlin's family.

Sara Carlin's tragic death was due to a blockbuster with a poor safety record, off-label prescribing, inadequate safety warnings that doctors ignored, and adverse reaction data a Big Pharma company chose to hide. Oh, and it didn't work for many patients.

And no one went to jail.

Seven years later and little had changed.[9]

As many of Oakville's beautiful young people crowded into St. Matthew's Catholic Church for Sara Carlin's memorial service in June, I sat alone in my home office trying to understand: What could her doctors have been thinking? Or were they thinking at all? I also searched my soul. Had anything I had done to help make others safer made any difference at all? When will we stop killing the innocent with blockbuster drugs?

VANESSA MEANS BUTTERFLY.

There is a theory that we are so interconnected on this planet that a butterfly flapping its wings on one side of our world might move the air just enough to stir up the beginnings of a breeze and wind. By a chain of events that wind could lead to weather changes and a hurricane on the other side of the world. It is my fervent hope that the people who read this story of one beautiful, innocent victim of corporate greed, government laxity, and medical error will act to make others safe.

Could the death of a butterfly in Oakville, Ontario, trigger a hurricane of drug reform around the world? Sometimes I feel the beginning of a breeze.

Notes

1   This story was recounted in the *Globe and Mail* by Dr. Miriam Schuchman.

Chapter 2: "They Dish it Out Like Water"

1   The *Compendium of Pharmaceuticals and Specialties* lists most of the drugs sold in Canada and contains the official prescribing information (drug label) approved by Health Canada for each, including any safety warnings the drug companies have seen fit to put into writing.
2   Benjamin Franklin is credited with this statement.

Chapter 3: A Predictable Death

1   These are the same words that are on Vanessa's grave marker and appear before Chapter one in this book.
2   Dr. Joel Lexchin, CMAJ, March 15, 2005. Drug withdrawals from the Canadian Market for Safety Reasons, 1963–2004.
3   Dr. David Graham, Associate Director of Safety at the U.S. FDA, testified Nov. 18, 2004, before a Senate sub-committee that Vioxx had probably caused between 55,000 and 65,000 deaths due to heart attacks and strokes. "This estimate ranges from 88,000 to 139,000 Americans. Of these, 30-40 per cent probably died. For the survivors, their lives were changed forever." It has since been exposed that Vioxx maker Merck had evidence from clinical studies way back in 2000 that revealed Vioxx might be causing heart attacks and strokes. Instead of ordering a clinical study to find out for sure, Merck spent about $100 million in advertising to drive Vioxx use up to double blockbuster status—$2.4 billion. About 58,000 Americans died in the Vietnam War.

4   After many hours of research I learned that SIDS is not a disease. It's not even a cause of a disease. It is more like a category in which coroners place infant deaths when they don't know what caused their deaths. SIDS is a catch-all for crib deaths when they have ruled everything else out. You can imagine it gave me little comfort to discover at this point that hundreds of babies die in their cribs every year and no one really knows why.

5   Jeremy Taylor is not his real name. His role is important to the legal side of my story, but his name is not. I have changed his name to avoid any legal wrangles that could result from my using his real name.

6   The unofficial keeper of the lists of drugs that might cause long QT, torsades de pointes, and heart arrhythmia with or without grapefruit juice is Dr. Ray Woosley at the University of Arizona CERT (Centers for Education and Research on Therapeutics). At their website the drugs can be searched by brand and generic names.

7   To this day I still don't know. Motilium (domperidone) is on University of Arizona CERT's list of drugs known to be a risk of long QT and torsades de pointes under certain circumstances. In fact it has never been approved in the U.S. However, Johnson & Johnson are selling it now off-label in Canada and in other countries—for one its side effects; under some circumstances Motilium initiates lactation. So an attempted revival of Motilium's fortunes is in process. In January 2006 Health Canada issued a new warning for domperidone for heart arrhythmias in the Adverse Reactions Newsletter—which most doctors never see. Over six years after Vanessa died and nothing significant had changed at Health Canada.

8   IMS Health Inc. is a $5 billion company that bills itself on its website as the "premier source of global pharmaceutical market intelligence."

9   It is unclear whether in Canada IMS tracks individual prescribing information by doctor today, or if it is more often by clinic or geographical area. In the U.S., individual tracking is the norm.

10 If doctors did track drugs by patient name on a spreadsheet they could quickly call all their patients about any drug that had raised safety concerns. Dr. Kayner later revealed that it took his staff weeks to call his patients on Prepulsid to warn them because they had to go through every individual patient file. The industry uses

database technology very creatively to help make sales and profits, but not to make patients safer.

11 I assume by "we" Dr. Eggar was referring a group of doctors at Oakville Trafalgar Memorial Hospital who had either formally or informally conducted a post-mortem discussion about Vanessa's death. I do know that Prepulsid was taken off the hospital formulary (no longer given to patients) within weeks.

Chapter 4: A Conspiracy of Silence

1 Alex Demerse is not his real name. Alex spoke to me candidly to help me understand how Vanessa had died and in fact why. His honesty was crucial for me to understand that. Unfortunately the nature of business is that using his real name could easily make him unemployable. I don't think it would be fair or that it's necessary for me to expose Alex to that risk. Alex is one of a handful people in this book who helped me along my journey that I do not name, and it's for the same reason in each case. I call them my angels. Without them this book would not exist.

2 The largest study on adverse drug reactions was done by Jason Lazarou and others, "Incidence of Adverse Drug Reactions in Hospitalized Patients," and reported in the *Journal of the American Medical Association* Vol. 279, No. 15 (April 15, 1998), pp. 1200-1205. The authors concluded that there were 106,000 deaths a year in U.S. hospitals from adverse drug reactions—caused by drugs taken as prescribed. This did not include accidental overdoses or drugs taken in error, estimated to cause another 100,000 deaths a year in the U.S. The estimated U.S. number of serious adverse drug reactions was over two million a year. No comparative studies have been done in Canada to my knowledge. But at approximately 10 per cent of the U.S. population, the Canadian population likely suffers 200,000 serious adverse drug reactions a year and 10,000 deaths from non-error prescriptions, and another possible 10,000 due to errors. In 1998 Canadian doctors only reported 1,265 serious adverse drug reactions (CMAJ April 6, 1999)—less than 1 per cent. ADR reports from all sources were 4,663. Health Canada officials try to maintain that 10 per cent of all ADRs are reported in Canada. It certainly makes them look

better. But outside of drug safety advocates I work with no family doctor I've spoken to reports them.

Chapter 5: They Knew, and They Didn't Tell

1   The official prescribing information is also known as the monograph or "label." It is the documentation approved by our regulators when they approve a drug. The label can be anywhere from eight to fifty pages long, the length being another reason doctors don't read labels. Patients rarely see drug labels.

2   I later discovered that this warning was provided after it was discovered that President Bill Clinton had been taking Prepulsid with omeprazole (Prilosec) for gastroesophageal reflux. One can imagine the discussions that took place amongst White House officials when it was discovered that Prepulsid, if taken with certain antibiotics, antifungals, or various other drugs could possibly have put the U.S. president at risk. But Clinton would not have been the first president to suffer an adverse reaction to a drug. President George Bush was seen on the TV news a few years before throwing up and almost falling face-first into his soup at a Japanese state dinner after taking Halcion. Abraham Lincoln suffered terrible side effects including fits of rage and gloom until in 1861, when he stopped taking a popular drug at the time for constipation, mercury—a poison.

3   Donald Rumsfeld is also the former chair of Gilead Sciences, creators of the flu drug Tamiflu. I suppose he would have understood the Prepulsid label.

4   This list of drugs that could be dangerous with Prepulsid has continued to grow. In August 2007, the website Drug.com listed 525 individual drugs that could cause interactions with Prepulsid and ninety-seven that could cause moderate reactions. It also reads: "Because a significant interaction may occur with red wine in the occasional patient, red wine should preferably be avoided also during cisapride therapy." My question is how long will this list get before Johnson & Johnson take Prepulsid off the world market?

Chapter 6: All Drugs Cause Adverse Effects

1   Ralph Nader also ran for U.S. president in 2000 and co-founded over twenty public interest groups in the U.S. He took on the auto industry with his book *Unsafe at any Speed* exposing the dangers of the Chevy Corvair. It is due largely to Ralph Nader's efforts that the auto industry now takes more responsibility for its customer's safety.

2   *Worst Pills–Best Pills*, Sidney Wolfe M.D. and Larry Sasich Ph.D., Pharm. Published in 1990, 1993, and 1999. I highly recommend this drug manual to you. It is one of the few places you will see prescription drug information that is not influenced by Big Pharma. This manual could save your life.

3   Lazarou et al.

4   See "Taking Care of Business," by Jenny Manzer, The *Ottawa Citizen*, December 21, 2006, p. A12; part of an important series of articles entitled "The Painful Truth," started December 19, 2006 in the same paper.

5   The U.S. Medwatch reporting system is voluntary, but a lot of U.S. patients use it. In 2005 Health Canada finally enabled their website to provide limited reported information on adverse drug reactions after the CBC had embarrassed them into it by doing so first.

6   The number of hospitals in Canada is now about 500 and the U.S. Census says there are over 8,000 total in the U.S. But there are also over two million patients in 20,000 long-term care facilities and nursing homes, mostly ailing seniors on multiple medications. Seniors were a large patient group for Prepulsid, especially those confined to a hospital bed.

Chapter 7: "Sleeping on the Yellow Line"

1   That appeal was heard by three judges in the Court of Appeal for Ontario in November 2000, who reduced the jury award of $50,000 to the victim's younger sister for guidance, care, and companionship to $25,000, despite her "very significant loss" and "a very close relationship."

2   Even nine-month-old Gage Steven's death in Pittsburgh was linked to Prepulsid along with Tagamet (cimetidine)—not a "clean" death.

3   And in time five hundred class actions as well—for an eventual total of 16,000 plaintiffs.

4   These kinds of tactics were not new to the medical profession, or to women. Dr. Gideon Koren at Sick Children's Hospital in Toronto sent out poison-pen letters about colleague Dr. Nancy Olivieri who was in conflict with a drug company. He was later identified by DNA evidence.

Chapter 8: A Message in a Bottle

1   I use the term whistleblower with the greatest respect. Some people feel it has gained a derogatory meaning related to those who blow the whistle on unsafe or illegal practices at their place of employment for money. A better term for people like Michele and Sana, who have not gained from speaking out, is "public guardian." I agree and use whistleblower here because it is a familiar term.

2   Canadian Adverse Drug Reaction Newsletter Volume 10, Number 1, January 2000.

3   One of the deaths was blamed on SIDS, which is not a cause of anything. Rather, as Gage Stevens' parents had tragically learned, under numerous conditions Prepulsid could be the cause of a SIDS death.

4   This might sound like an unfair characterization. But Janssen-Ortho officials had sent documents stating their official position on Prepulsid to Health Canada officials in advance of public release on another occasion and coached them on how to handle difficult questions about Prepulsid, including what "angles" to take with the media. Filmmaker Erna Buffie had obtained a number of Health Canada documents through the Freedom of Information Act. One of them was a fax of Janssen's Media Standby Statement sent by Alain Raoult, vice-president, Scientific Affairs, to Dr. Chris Turner at Health Canada the day after the CBC broadcast about Prepulsid on November 2, 1999. It included a handwritten note to Dr. Turner saying "feel free to call me" with his office and home telephone number. An internal email to Dr. Turner from Dr. Agnes Klein dated 99/08/11 summarized the Prepulsid label changes since 1995. It advises Dr. Turner: "Alain is quite happy to provide any information or clarification you need. He believes the 'angle' is that 'voluntary' reporting does not work; that he declined the interview

because it was *NOT LIVE*; [Dr. Klein's italics] that changes to 'labeling' of drugs is a progressive task as knowledge advances; that timing between US and Canada cannot always be the same due to differences in the two systems . . ." So Janssen executives were not only telling Health Canada officials what to say about Prepulsid, but how to say it! Is it any wonder Prepulsid stayed on the market despite having so many dangerous contraindications?

5 National Institutes of Health (NIH) is one of the world's foremost medical research centres—a U.S. government agency. AZT is an AIDS drug that was proving to be effective in treating AIDS.

6 Note this has changed under The Federal Accountability Act, adopted January 1, 2007.

7 Michele was right. The Motilium patent ran out just after Johnson & Johnson introduced Prepulsid.

8 Hoechst Marion Roussel makes Seldane, Seldane D, Allegra, and Allegra D. Seldane was withdrawn in December 1997 about the time Allegra D was approved by the FDA. Allegra was approved in Canada in June 1997.

9 This conversation took place in 2000. In April 2008 the federal government introduced amendments to the Food and Drugs Act that will provide Health Canada officials with the direct authority to pull prescription drugs and other health products off the market, rather than advising the Minister to do so.

10 Up until Vioxx in 2004, thalidomide was the worst drug disaster in history. Thalidomide was sold in the sixties to expectant mothers as being very safe, to combat morning sickness. Thousands of deformed infants were born worldwide in the late fifties and sixties to mothers who took the drug. Thousands of others died shortly after birth. West German drugmaker Grunenthal claimed it was safe and effective until the day it was pulled off the market.

Chapter 9: And Man Created Blockbuster

1 From the Dermatologists.ca website: Dr. Shear was also a professor & Chief of Dermatology at the University of Toronto Medical School. He had published 200 peer-reviewed papers and numerous chapters and abstracts. In 1997 CADRAC morphed into Health Canada's Expert Advisory Committee on Pharmacovigilance, on which Neil serves.

2   IMS Health is the $5 billion company that collects and sells information on pharmaceuticals worldwide.

3   Dr. Alan Kaplan is a professor of psychiatry, head of Toronto General Hospital's eating disorders program and president of the International Academy for Eating Disorders. He was the first holder of the Canadian-endowed chair in Eating Disorders at University of Toronto in 2002.

4   Michele was right. The Canadian Food and Drugs Act states; Section C.08.006. 16-8-95 (2) "The Minister may, by notice to a manufacturer, suspend, for a definite or indefinite period, a notice of compliance issued to that manufacturer in respect of a new drug submission or an abbreviated new drug submission or a supplement to either submission, if the Minister considers (a) that the drug is not safe for the use represented in the submission or supplement, as shown by evidence obtained from (i) clinical or other experience not reported in the submission or supplement or not available to the Minister at the time the notice of compliance was issued." To pull a drug off the market, Health Canada officials need only to advise the Minister of Health to withdraw a notice of compliance, because the drug can no longer be prescribed safely. Any Minister refusing to take that advice could be accepting personal ethical responsibility for potential injuries and deaths of patients, and taking considerable political risk. Based on my experience in government, with a drug like Prepulsid, bureaucratic advice to withdraw the notice of compliance would be automatically followed by the Minister of Health. So lack of direct bureaucratic authority to order a drug off the market with cause is in my view an excuse for inaction. In April 2008, the Harper government introduced amendments to the Food and Drugs Act to give bureaucrats direct authority to pull an unsafe drug off the market.

5   Johnson & Johnson markets a group of drugs that all end in the suffix "azole." [Some "azole" drugs are made by other companies.] They are drugs that people take orally to fight a fungus in their bloodstream. These drugs, along with Prepulsid are broken down (metabolized) by the same group of enzymes in our system, called P450 CYP3A4. They are all—or should all—be contraindicated for each other, i.e. all the "azole" drugs are contraindicated for Prepulsid and grapefruit juice, because the combination can cause

heart arrhythmia if the patient's body can't break Prepulsid down and clear it properly. The drug then builds up to a level in the blood that is dangerous. When that happens the heart can go into arrhythmia and stop. None of this affected Vanessa because she was taking no other drug. Prepulsid was also dangerous on its own.

6   *JAMA.* 1998;279:1200-1205. The estimated figure was 106,000 U.S. deaths a year in hospitals. Canada's population is about 10 per cent of the U.S. population. That means that probably over 10,000 Canadians die a year from adverse drug reactions in hospitals taking prescription drugs as prescribed. Some experts believe another 10,000 Canadians die from adverse drug reactions outside hospitals, including prescribing errors, errors in administration of the drug, and accidental overdoses.

7   Ibid. The researchers estimated that in 1994 overall 2,216,000 (1,721,000–2,711,000) hospitalized patients had serious ADRs and 106,000 (76,000–137,000) had fatal ADRs, making these reactions between the fourth- and sixth-leading cause of death.

8   This story was told on CBC's *Marketplace* program, produced by Rene Pellerin in November 1999.

9   Alan is co-author of *Selling Sickness*, with Ray Moynihan, one of my sources for this book that I recommend to you. (*Selling Sickness, How the World's Biggest Pharmaceutical Companies Are Turning Us All into Patients.* Ray Moynihan, Alan Cassels. Grey Stone Books, 2005.)

10 *Bitter Pills*, Fried, Stephen. Bantam Books, May 1999 p. 244.

11 Ibid. p. 245.

12 "The pharmaceutical Industry—To Whom is it Accountable?" Angell, M. *New England Journal of Medicine*, June 22, 2000.

13 Rx&D, the Big Pharma lobby in Canada, are constantly reminding our politicians that the Big Pharma jobs in Canada are conditional upon our governments supporting their industry. In April 2006 the chair of Rx&D, Paul Lucas, told the Mississauga Chamber of Commerce that industry jobs and economic spinoffs—on "pill hill" where GlaxoSmithKline and others have plants, were under threat, because the Ontario government was introducing changes to its prescription drug formulary rules: "Indeed, many countries are now actively competing to attract the innovative pharmaceutical industry and its R&D. Countries like the U.S., Singapore, Ireland, India,

and China, and the province of Quebec. But make no mistake, if the Ministry's policy moves forward unchanged, over time, 'Pill Hill' will deteriorate. In 10 or 15 years, you won't be hearing about the wonderful R&D successes in Mississauga, you will be hearing about these discoveries happening in other countries. The government now has a very clear choice to make." Lucas compared Big Pharma's Ontario portion of the total 8.8 per cent of Canadian sales Rx&D spend on research and development to the historical loss of the Avro Arrow and its impact on the Canadian aerospace industry—quite a stretch.

14 When a new president took over, Gilmartin was made Special Advisor to the Board.

Chapter 10: This Business of Disease

1 Omeprazole (Losec) was a purple pill, as is Nexium. "The purple pill" is a marketing term AstraZeneca used to promote Nexium, now a multiple blockbuster.

2 Families USA Report 2001.

3 AFL-CIO web page "Executive Paywatch Database," http://www.aflcio.org/corporatewatch/paywatch/ceou/database.cfm

4 March 17, 2000. Press Release, Representative Carolyn Maloney: "Maloney to Drug Companies: Enough is Enough" www.maloney.house.gov

5 Associated Press, December 21, 2006. Hank's goodbye present from Pfizer shareholders "included an estimated $82.3 million in pension benefits, $77.9 million in deferred compensation, and cash and stock totaling more than $20.7 million. The total value could grow to almost $200 million if McKinnell gets a $19.3 million stock award, but that is contingent on the future performance of the stock of the world's largest drug maker."

6 November 8, 2002, *The Romanow Commission on the Future of Healthcare in Canada, Final Report*, p. 194.

7 Ibid. p. 194 quoting a study published in *Geriatrics Today* in 2001 by Kidney and MacKinnon.

8 Drug-Related Hospitalizations in a Tertiary Care. Internal Medicine Service of a Canadian Hospital: A Prospective Study, Leslie Jo Samoy et al. Pharmacotherapy 2006:26(11):1578–1586. The study excluded admissions for pediatric care, surgery, coronary care,

intensive care, obstetrical and gynecological care, and psychiatric care. Out of 565 admissions 136 were drug related. 8.4 per cent (48) were adverse drug reactions; 4.2 per cent (24) were related to an inappropriate drug, 3.8 per cent (22) were due to noncompliance. Seventy per cent of the admissions were thought to be preventable.

9   Joel Lexchin also wrote the book Alan Cassels had read, *The Real Pushers: A Critical Analysis of the Canadian Drug Industry*, Vancouver: New Star Books, 1984.

10 "Do higher drug costs lead to better health?" *Canadian Journal of Clinical Pharmacology* Vol 12 (1) Winter 2005; e22 January 7, 2005, quoting PMPRB reports.

11 *JAMA* 2000;284:3036-3039. "Contraindicated Use of Cisapride, Impact of Food and Drug Administration Regulatory Action" Smalley et al.

12 Actually for most people there is a cheap safe way to lower high cholesterol: regular exercise, diet change and eating a handful of almonds every day. Did your doctor recommend that?

13 New Internationalist on-line magazine. Issue 362, Big Pharma Facts. Referencing Rachel Cohen, "An Epidemic of Neglect: Neglected diseases and the health burden in poor countries," Multinational Monitor, Vol 23. no 6. June 2002.

14 Ibid. p. 12.

15 Higher-than-average cholesterol is not a disease. It is a risk factor for heart disease. But so are about 200 *other* risk factors like being overweight, smoking, stress, and creased ear lobes. Men with creased ear lobes have a greater risk for heart disease than others. Why? No one knows. Since Big Pharma have pills to lower cholesterol—statins—that's the risk factor you hear about. Statins can sometimes cause some dreadful side effects.

16 In 1983 the U.S. government passed the Orphan Drug Act which provides tax deductions, better patent rules and other help to companies that produce orphan drugs. Since that time 249 orphan drugs have been given marketing authorization in the U.S. "including drugs to treat glioma, multiple myeloma, cystic fibrosis and snake venom." Simply put, without U.S. government action, there would have been no drugs for these illnesses. This is a superb example of how government can be a force for good, and if there's no money in it, Big Pharma is generally not interested.

17 Celebrex remains on the market for now, although Public Citizen put it on their "Do Not Use" list because safer alternatives are available like aspirin and ibuprofen. It may be off the market by the time you read this book. Mobic (meloxicam) is another drug on Public Citizen's "Do Not Use" Cox-2 group.

18 In January 2007 Johnson & Johnson and Health Canada were up to their old tricks again. It turns out that domperidone can cause heart arrhythmias like Prepulsid when taken orally as well, and sometimes it causes long QT and torsade de pointes. Sound familiar? So how did Johnson & Johnson and Health Canada warn new mothers? Déjà vu. An article was put in the Adverse Reaction Newsletter—the one that few doctors read.

19 "Pfizer gives up testing Viagra on Women," The *New York Times*, by Gardiner Harris. February 24, 2004. "... arousal and desire are often disconnected in women, the researchers found, to their consternation." Comedian Billy Crystal puts it differently: "Women need a reason to have sex. Men just need a place."

20 Winds of Change.net, Sufi Wisdom: The Camel and the Tent. Thanks to T.L. James who wrote this July 16, 2005 on Marsblog. adapted from an old Sufi tale: One cold night a Bedouin's camel woke him up. "Master, it is cold. May I put my nose inside the tent to warm it?" The traveller agreed. A short time later the camel woke him again. "It is cold. Can I put my head inside the tent?" First his head was admitted to the tent, then, on the same argument, his neck. Finally, without asking, the camel heaved his whole bulk under the cloth. The tent hung dangling across his hump. The Bedouin was lying beside the camel, with no protection from the cold.

Chapter 11: Deny. Delay. Divide. Discredit.

1 I never saw evidence of any financial relationship between Janssen-Ortho and three of the doctors that saw Vanessa. The gastroenterologist did have a previous financial relationship with the Janssen-Ortho—a research award. Dr. Kayner testified he met with drug reps in his office.

2 We included the College of Pharmacists because they set the standards of practice for dispensing prescription drugs, which includes the duty

of pharmacists to enter into a dialogue with patients when a drug may produce a side effect—another warning Vanessa never got.

3   In civil trials the standard of proof is "on the balance of probabilities." In criminal trials because the sanctions are so high—prison sentences—the standard is higher: "beyond a reasonable doubt." But with adverse drug reactions the industry and our regulators want "cause and effect"—a standard that is a virtual certainty. This is a key reason dangerous drugs are left on the market. Cause and effect is a ridiculously high standard of proof. It is folly to apply a laboratory standard to public safety. Our regulators should unilaterally adopt a new standard of proof for ADRs: association. If they can prove a drug is associated with serious ADRs they should immediately issue clear warnings, or with a pattern of them, withdraw the drug. Big Pharma will fight this I suspect to their last breath.

4   Seldane was not a Johnson & Johnson drug.

5   Ray is now at the University of Arizona. The list of drugs can be found at the university website under CERT.

6   Interview with Dr. Paul Janssen. D Healy (Ed.) The Psychopharmacologists. London: Altman, 1998.

7   A similar warning was issued in Canada in March 2001, three years later.

8   Between 1997 and 1998 three fast-track drugs had been pulled off the U.S. market for injuring and killing patients. Faster approvals means less scrutiny, more people taking them, and greater risk for patients. With truly breakthrough drugs that might make sense. But 95% of new drugs aren't significantly new treatments. Big Pharma wants to make money faster, so they promise to do safety studies AFTER you and your family members start taking them. They are Health Canada's "partners."

9   CMAJ August 3, 2004 171 (3) "New Directions in Drug approval," Dr. Joel Lexchin Quoting Dr. Chris Turner, Director General of the Marketed Health Products Directorate at that time.

10   CMAJ, March 15, 2005 "Drug Withdrawals from the Canadian market for safety reasons," 1963-2004 Joel Lexchin.

Chapter 12; Games with Names

1   *Corporate Crime in the Pharmaceutical Industry*, Braithwaite, John. London: Routledge & Kegan Paul, 1984. p. 66.

2   *Corporate Crime in the Pharmaceutical Industry* p. 65-66 and PEDIATRICS Vol. 110 No. 2 August 2002, pp. 404-406. The confusion of brand names delayed the embargo in some countries; for example, authorities in Brazil "seized two and a half million pills 6 months after the withdrawal in Germany, along with another 100 tons" of the drug in bulk form. "In Italy and in Japan thalidomide remained on the market for . . . 9 months" after the withdrawal in Germany.

3   Health Canada started to put adverse drug reaction reports on their website after a number of stories the CBC broadcast on unsafe drugs including Vanessa's, and after the CBC embarrassed them into it allowing consumers to report adverse drug reactions on their website. It was a journalist in Brazil who first alerted the public in Brazil to the dangers of thalidomide.

4   There are at least three names under which cisapride is sold in India.

5   U.S. Food and drug Administration web page, *FDA Consumer Magazine*, July-August 2005 Issue. Author Carol Rados.

6   January-February 2004, *Journal of the American Pharmacists Association*.

7   A study of four clinical drug trials and six studies (called meta-analyses) published in March 2006 from the New Zealand Medical Research Institute showed that Celebrex (celecoxib) may double the risk for heart attacks compared to older arthritis drugs.

8   Drug Discovery Ltd. Vol. 5, No. 7 July 2000, Alan Harvey, Strategies for discovering drugs from previously unexplored natural products; referenced from J. Nat. Prod. 60. 52-60 by G.M. Cragg et al. (1977) Natural Products in drug discovery and development.

9   *New York Times*, December 27, 2003, "The Science of Naming Drugs," by Donald G. McNeil Jr. as reprinted on igorinternational.com

10   PMDD stands for Premenstrual Dysphoric Disorder. It one of many disorders identified in recent years by *The Diagnostic and Statistical Manual of Mental Disorders*. Psychiatrists do not all agree that PMDD is a disease. It refers to mood swings that some women suffer one or two weeks before their period. Some psychiatrists

believe PMDD is a normal part of life that is inappropriate for drug therapy treatment. Prozac has potential side effects that can cause worse symptoms than those caused be PMDD. Dr. David Healy. author of *Let Them Eat Prozac*, believes 25,000 people have committed suicide due to Prozac in the last thirty years that would not otherwise have done so.

11 Thioridazine is Mellaril, a Novartis antipsychotic drug prescribed for schizophrenic patients. It was taken off the market in Canada in September 2005, and the FDA ordered a black box warning be placed on the U.S. drug label in July 2000. It can cause long QT and heart arrhythmia, especially with other drugs. The Prozac warning also tells doctors that even adult patients "should be watched closely." I've never seen a doctor that has time to do that. And many people live alone, with no one to watch them at home.

12 Comedian Jerry Seinfeld on over-the-counter drugs: "Some people aren't satisfied with extra, [strength] they want maximum! 'Gimme the maximum strength! Give the maximum allowable human dosage! That's the kind of pain I'm in! Figure out what will kill me, and then back it off a little bit.'" But what is a safe dose for most people may be dangerous for some.

13 FDA Medwatch, FDA Drug Safety Page, October 7, 2002. See the FDA/CDER website.

14 *National Post*. November 13, 2006. "Drug Names Confusion risks lives of Canadians," Tom Blackwell.

15 Scoop Independent News, March 20, 2006. Evelyn Pringle. "Just what Kids need—Sparlon—another ADHA Drug." These adverse reactions were reported during clinical studies for Sparlon.

Chapter 13: Do No Harm

1 Journalist David Willman won a Pulitzer Prize for the articles in 2001.

2 A Government of Canada interdepartmental working group identified these five historic pillars of public policy and considerations regarding drug policy.

3 Dr. Michele Brill-Edwards was obliged to quit after a senior manager she had gone to a judge about this (and had been fired,) was re-hired by Health Canada.

4   I believe if these people—who worked in the branch that reviewed animal vaccines—were in charge of the safety of Prepulsid, Vanessa would be alive today. So on May 9, 2005, under the auspices of Drug Safety Canada I created The Vanessa Young Award, for public guardians who show integrity and courage in public service. Their right to dissent honestly in the public interest without retaliation has since been confirmed by the federal court. These four and four others—Dr. Michele Brill-Edwards, Nicholas Regush, Pierre Blais and Dr. Nancy Olivieri were recognized as "public guardians" at a ceremony in Ottawa hosted by the Canadian Health Coalition.

5   Public Policy Forum document, "Improving Canada's Regulatory Process for Therapeutic Products," Spring 2003 Section 1.

6   When the media is there, they are "spun." But when the media is not there, the results can be spun beyond all recognition.

7   Government of Canada, Department of Finance 2003 Budget Document. "Building the Canada we want: Investing in Canada's health care system."

8   "Improving Canada's Regulatory Process for Therapeutic Products," Public Policy Forum Spring 2003 Newsletter, p. 3. What impact will this deliberation have?

9   Naturally I later wrote to Health Canada officials and told them I would not be attending their "plenary" session, which would bring us together with three other groups: Big Pharma reps, "disease awareness" groups (many financed in part by Big Pharma) and healthcare professionals—many of whom I knew were on the Big Pharma money bandwagon. If we couldn't even get our concerns written down honestly at the session for public interest groups, I could imagine what kind of final document PPF would produce with this huge pharma influence. I couldn't lend my own credibility or the organization I had founded—Drug Safety Canada to a process dominated by drug industry influence and positioned to bring forward their agenda.

10 Public Policy Forum, Concluding Report from the Multi-Stakeholder Session June 25-26, 2003, Fairmont Chateau Laurier, Ottawa, Ontario, p. 6. Seven Critical Directions for Action. This statement is another good example of bureaucratic-speak—virtually meaningless.

Chapter 14: Physician, Heal Thyself

1   January 2, 2001, the *Globe and Mail*, "Drug Firm's Freebies entice doctors: Debate raging in medical community over pharmaceutical marketing practices." Krista Foss.

2   Drug labels as printed in the *CPS* use fewer pages because the print is so tiny. On the Internet I've seen labels over 50 pages.

3   World Health Organization, International Conferences on Improving Use of Medicines, "How does pharmaceutical company promotion affect prescribing?" reprinted from *Scrip Magazine*, March 1995. P.R. Mansfield.

4   Ibid.

5   Mike's story is told by researcher and writer Alan Cassels in *Common Ground*, "Donuts for Doctors" Sept. 2005. Kathleen Slattery-Moschkau is a former sales representative for Bristol-Myers Squibb and Johnson & Johnson who also left the industry. She has produced the film "Side Effects" which looks at the pharmaceutical business from the inside. See also *Prescription Games*, Robinson, Jeffery, McClelland & Stewart Limited, p. 203 on detail rep personal databases.

6   Medical Anthropology Q 18:328-356 Oldani, Mike (2004) Thick prescriptions: Toward an interpretation of pharmaceutical sales practices. Taken from the PLoS Medicine website. Following the Script: How Drug Reps Make Friends and Influence Doctors. Adriane Fugh-Berman, Shahram Ahari. Shahram Ahari is a former Eli Lilly drug detail rep.

7   *Atlantic Monthly*, April 2006, Elliot C. The Drug Pushers. Ibid. PloS Medicine website article.

8   Ibid. Medical Anthropology Q 18: 328-356 Oldani, Mike (2004) Thick Prescriptions.

9   PLoS Medicine website. Following the Script: How Drug Reps Make Friends and Influence Doctors. Adriane Fugh-Berman, Shahram Ahari.

10 I say "many" because there are drug reps that don't believe what they are saying, and know very well their drugs cause serious adverse drug reactions they never tell the doctors about. They either don't care, or find it difficult to leave the business. I spent a lot of time on websites where drug reps chat anonymously to each other.

Their comments about risky drugs and sleazy marketing are very revealing. Frankly, many of the reps on the chat sites are not the kind of people you would want your doctor even meeting with. Check out www.cafepharma.com, click Boards, then Company Boards and pick a drug company. It's funny sometimes, as you can spot where a pharma PR shill has logged on anonymously to slip in the party line. As with many things on the Internet one can't prove the comments are written by drug detail reps or pharma PR people, but the pharma-speak they use and easy familiarity with the drugs is convincing. Log on and decide for yourself.

11 *JAMA* "The Accuracy of drug information from pharmaceutical sales representatives," Zeigler et al., *JAMA* 273:1296-1298.

12 Chren, MM, Landefeld, CS. "Physicians' behavior and their interactions with drug companies: a controlled study of physicians who requested additions to a hospital drug formulary." *JAMA*. 1994;271,684-689.

13 Prescription Games, (ibid.) p. 198 Quoting a career brochure from Merck.

14 US FDA Consumer Magazine online July-August 2004 Issue. "Drug Maker to Pay $430 Million in Fines, Civil Damages."

15 Generation RX (ibid.) p. 104. I am indebted to Greg Critser for his work on this excellent book which I recommend to you.

16 Generation RX (ibid.) p. 105.

17 *San Francisco Chronicle*, May 14, 2004, Huge penalty in drug fraud. Bernadette Tansey.

18 *San Francisco Chronicle*, May 1, 2005. Hard Sell, How Marketing Drives the Pharmaceutical Industry, Bernadette Tansey.

Chapter 15: Get 'em While They're Young

1   As of August 2007 there were 476 serious ADRs related to Duragesic on the Health Canada website with 91 related deaths, most often with other drugs involved. However, since most adverse drug reactions are not reported, this likely means thousands of serious ADRs and additional related deaths may have never been reported. Warning: Health Canada inexplicably insist on identifying ADRs reported related to an active ingredient under their various names. So someone looking under Duragesic might miss checking fentanyl—

the active ingredient—and underestimate the reports and risks. I found an additional 217 ADR reports for fentanyl, Ran-fentanyl and Ratio-fentanyl—by checking all the names, and another ten related deaths. If you truly wanted to warn doctors and patients about fentanyl wouldn't you report them all in the same place? In September 2005 Janssen-Ortho issued a Public Advisory regarding possible overdose with Duragesic, saying among other things, "There have been reports of deaths in children using Duragesic in Canada." The public is supposed to guess if the reports are accurate or not.

2   This practice has been going on for decades. Drug reps inside medical schools look for ways to ingratiate themselves with the future gatekeepers for their products. However, there are some doctors who are working to put a stop to it. They know that the debts of gratitude affect prescribing behaviour and that this is highly inappropriate. Some medical schools have established policies prohibiting drug company sales representatives in some circumstances. Check out some fascinating stories at the website www.nofreelunch.org.

3   I later discovered a study from *The Journal of the American Medical Association* (Sept 7, 2005). Over 800 U.S. medical students were surveyed and 93.2 per cent said they had been asked or required by a doctor to attend a free lunch paid for by Big Pharma. By third year the students reported they got one gift or attended one drug company sponsored event a week. 68.8 per cent of them report that the gifts would not influence their prescribing. "80 per cent of students say they believe they are entitled to the gifts." Source: Eyeforpharma on-line pharma marketing website. My question is: how does Big Pharma get the names of the students before classes start?

4   Hundreds of lawsuits have been settled or litigated against American Home Products Corporation, the company that marketed the diet drug fen-phen, for causing heart valve damage.

5   *Basic and Applied Psychology* 1997, Vol 19, NO. 1, pp. 91-100, "Effects on Time on the Norm of Reciprocity," Burger et al.

6   University of Alberta, Rounds News, Feb. 23/2006 "Physician and Industry Interactions: How well do we mix?" J. de Bruyn et al.

7   The increased prescriptions of the brand drugs included "making formulary requests for medications that rarely held important advantages over existing ones," and "prescribing fewer generic but

more expensive, newer medications at no demonstrated advantage." My question is: Why else would the companies spend the money?

8   *British Medical Journal*, 2003;326:1199-1192 (31 May) "Who pays for the pizza? Redefining the relationships between doctors and drug companies. Part 1. Entanglement" Ray Moynihan.

9   *Med Market Media* 40: 96. Marshall PC (2005) "Rep tide: Pulling back in magnitude, pushing forward efficiency: Recent talk of pharma companies restructuring or even paring back their sales forces is the first acknowledgement that efficiency, and not noise, is the key to effective detailing." Taken from PloS Medicine website: Following the Script: How Drug Reps Make Friends and Influence Doctors, Adriane Fugh-Berman, Shahram Ahari.

10 www.PharmaceuticalRepTraining.com Homepage "There are approximately 625,000 physicians" in the U.S., and "Of those 625,000 physicians about 125,000 are high-volume prescribers." Canada has an additional 57,000 practicing physicians—total 682,000.

11 Blumenthal, D. "Doctors and Drug Companies." *NEJM* 2004;351 (19) The *Globe and Mail* story in January 2001 written by Krista Foss estimated $20,000/year per doctor on all marketing efforts.

12 *Prescription Games* (ibid.) p. 195.

13 Ibid.

14 *Humanist Perspectives*, Issue 153, "The Buying of the Medical Profession," by Alan Cassels. p. 5.

15 Lemmens, *CMAJ* 1998.

16 Katx, *American Journal of Bioethics* 2003.

17 Ethics, *Journal of the American Medical Association*, June 2006, V 8. Number 6, p. 413 "Firms that manufacture FDA-regulated products (primarily pharmaceuticals) provided three quarters (74.7 per cent) of the income of medical education and communications companies (MECCs)" These are the companies that operate CME events.

18 Until 2005 the Rx&D website listed these infractions of the pharma "voluntary" code of ethics going back years on its website. AstraZeneca seemed to get caught the most. The maximum fine for infractions of the Code of Conduct was apparently $15,000. I have written twice to Rx&D via their website to ask why this information is not longer made available on their website with no reply.

19 Personal email correspondence from Alan Cassels, Researcher with The University of Victoria, Canada, and co-author of *Selling Sickness*.

Chapter 16: Ganging Up on Vanessa

1 Letter from the FDA to Cynthia Chianese, Assistant Director, Regulatory Affairs, Janssen Pharmaceutica, Titusville, NJ, USA. Time-stamped June 4, 1998.

2 Brand name Zantac, a drug that reduces stomach acid.

3 I do not know if the lawyer from Health Canada or the pharmacists went to dinner with the others. In fact I don't know 100% if that planned dinner happened. But it seemed clear to me over the next few days by the questions that there was a concerted effort from all sides to fault Vanessa. It was not pretty to see a bunch of grown men doing such a thing.

4 As did the Liberal and even some NDP politicians. Corporations in many industries buy tickets for party fundraisers. That has now been banned federally.

5 As you can imagine, as a lobbyist, I have never done any work for any pharma or tobacco interests.

6 Not every major drug company donates to politicians and parties directly in Canada. Sometimes they donate indirectly through their lobby group in Canada, Rx&D, or in the U.S.—PhRMA, www.phrma.org

7 Every year the TV news crews have gone out to shoot a few seconds of film at the big spring Conservative or Liberal "Heritage" Dinners—both provincially and federally. I chuckle when they use their cliché: "This evening, 2,000 well-heeled Conservatives (or Liberals) paid $500 a plate to hear party leader [whomever] speak . . ." The funny thing is, it's the major corporations—including Big Pharma—that buy those tables and send their people in to fill the seats. And to a large degree it's the same company people at *both* events, making sure they meet the key players and that those players know they are party contributors. Corporate donations have since been totally banned by the Harper government in 2007.

8 Of the sixteen drugs taken off the market since 1997, half were fast-track approvals that should never have been approved in the first place.

9 As of June 2007 the new federal limit to leadership contests is $1,100 total for individuals, with no corporate, business or union donations allowed. However, large loans to those who want to become Prime Minister are still allowed—such as the $720,000 loan to Liberal leadership candidate Bob Rae from his brother John, who is Executive Vice-President in the office of the Chairman of Power Corporation, one of Canada's most politically influential companies. It appears that Rae, a former NDP premier of Ontario, has gone corporate.

10 Hiring former politicians and current staff is not a practice limited to Big Pharma companies. These people have to work somewhere. But Big Pharma is a leader in "strategic" hiring.

11 By an amazing coincidence there has been a lot more Big Pharma investment in Quebec per capita than elsewhere in Canada.

12 National Post, February 3, 2004, From CanWest News Service Ottawa Citizen. Aide who advised Martin now lobbies him. Glen McGregor.

13 Ottawa Citizen, June 27, 2006. "Drug Firm's research spending falls short." By Glen McGregor.

14 CBC.ca News September 25, 2002. "More research for more patent protection: drug companies."

15 Toronto Star, June 5, 2006. "Premier on the spot over new drug bill," Ian Urquhart's column. The Ontario Ministry of Health documents refer to total Ontario government drug buying costs as $3.5 billion.

16 Unless the British High Commissioner just acted on his own. The letter was quoted: "The reforms introduced in Bill 102 will come at a steep price to the competitive attractiveness of the Ontario economy and to Ontario's reputation for reliability as an innovative partner." Some might feel that sending this letter to the Premier of Ontario at the behest of private industry is reminiscent of the days when Canada was a British colony. The UK is home to the head offices of two major pharmaceutical companies GlaxoSmithKline and AstraZeneca.

17 They delayed implementation of generic substitution until April 2007, and dropped therapeutic substitution altogether.

Chapter 17: Friends in Very High Places

1 Martha Murray's story is told in detail on the Internet at www.marthamurray.ca

2 Inquest into the Death of Vanessa Young, March 26, 2001, Hamilton, Ontario, Cross examination of Health Canada doctor by Gary Will.

3 The new Canada Health Protection Act was supposed to replace the Food and Drugs Act, The Radiation Emitting Devices Act, The Quarantine Act, and The Hazardous Products Act.

4 *Winnipeg Free Press*, December 26, 2003, "The fox is in the hen house." Frances Russell.

5 *Journal of Health Politics, Policy and Law*, V 28, Number 4, August 2003 pp. 615-658. Wiktorowicz, Mary E. "Emergent Patterns in the Regulation of Pharmaceuticals: Institutions and Interests in the United States, Canada, Britain and France." Referred from York University Press Release October 1, 2003 "Cheaper drug testing comes at a cost: York U. professor. Globalization lowers safety standards, increases public health risks."

6 Later, on January 28, 2004, an open letter was sent to Prime Minister Paul Martin asking among other things that he instruct the Minister of Health to adopt the precautionary principle for all risk assessment, and strictly enforce the ban on DTC advertising. It was signed by hundreds of individuals from twenty-seven countries including me for Drug Safety Canada. You can see the letter and who signed it at www.healthcoalition.ca

7 "Opening up the Medicine Cabinet," Report of the Standing Committee on Health. I testified for The Standing Committee on Health in Toronto at the King Edward Hotel Nov. 29, 2003 about what I had learned about Health Canada and the drug industry. That testimony is available on Hansard on the House of Commons website.

8 In the U.S. such information has been easily available on the Internet at Medline for years.

9 The Centre for Public Integrity Special Report Drug Lobby, "Second to None: How the pharmaceutical industry gets its way on Washington," July 7, 2005 by M. Asif Ismail.

10 U.S. citizens pay the highest prices in the world for their drugs. Canadians pay around the world median prices—about 40% below the U.S. This irks Big Pharma no end.

11 www.therubins.com, Crossing the Border to Obtain Cheaper Prescription Drugs-Part IV.

12 This is verified in the book *A Call to Action* written by Hank McKinnell, former CEO of Pfizer, where he said: "Drugs from Canadian pharmacies are as safe as drugs from pharmacies in the United States."

13 This one is still out there—about other countries. Never let it be said certain parties give up easily.

14 www.VOAnews.com Los Angeles, O'Sullivan Report, "Author describes intrigue behind The Karasik Conspiracy," Mike Sullivan.

15 *Boston Globe*, November 11, 2004 "Canada Threatens to Halt Shipments of Drugs to US." Christopher Rowland.

16 In 2005 Democratic House Leader Nancy Pelosi was quoted: "President Bush must stop serving as a handmaiden for the pharmaceutical industry." Source: *Detroit News* December 26th, 2004. Taken from Canada Drug Talk.com President G.W. Bush's father, the former President Bush, was on the Board of Directors of Eli Lilly before he was President and has been since he was defeated. Big Pharma companies are major donors to President Bush's campaigns and both the Republican and Democratic parties in the U.S.

Chapter 18: You Must Be Sick . . . Because They Need You to Be.

1 Inquest into the death of Vanessa Young, Coroner David Eden. April 2, 2001 Question 197.

2 Ibid. question 192.

3 Ibid. questions 294 & 295.

4 Ibid. question 114.

5 Ibid. question 243.

6 Inquest into the Death of Vanessa Young March 30, 2001, Testimony of Wendy Arnott. Question 38.

7 Ibid. Testimony of psychiatrist April 3, 2001 Q. 327.

8 Inquest into the Death of Vanessa Young, April 4, 2001. Testimony of psychiatrist Questions 29 and 31.

9 The following two sections, referring to the testimony of Doctors George Klein and Stuart MacLeod were sourced in my own notes taken at the time and the notes of Gary Will's assistant, law student Vanessa A. Tanner.

Chapter 19: There's No Such Thing as Monsters

1   Koerner C. US FDA Division of Drug Marketing, Advertising and Communications. Presentation at Health Canada Multi-Stakeholders' Consultation on Direct-to-Consumer Advertising. Aylmer, Quebec. April 14, 1999. Quoted from Health Action International and Canadian Health Coalition report, January 2004.

2   American Society of Newspaper Editors, August 10, 1999. "Perceived Bias." The study/poll report was titled "Examining our Credibility."

3   "Drugs in the news: an analysis of Canadian newspaper coverage of new prescription drugs." Alan Cassels, Merrilee A. Hughes, Carol Cole, Barbara Mintzes, Joel Lexchin, James P. McCormack. Get it at www.policyalternatives.ca

4   Ibid. Source: American society of Newspaper Editors.

5   Women who take Fosamax usually alter their lifestyle by quitting smoking, eating more foods with calcium, practicing better posture, and exercising more. It's possible the action of taking a pill daily also makes them more aware of winter ice, obstacles on the floor, and their surroundings—so they fall less. It might not even be the drug that's reducing broken hips!

6   "Fosamax Does More Harm Than Good," accessed September 3, 2007, lawyersandsettlements.com by Evelyn Pringle. "In a 2004 letter published in the Annals of Internal Medicine, researcher Susan Ott, MD, of the University of Washington wrote: 'Many people believe that these drugs are bone builders, but the evidence shows they are actually bone hardeners.'"

7   Canwest, whose assets include the Global TV network and the *National Post* newspaper, is asking the Ontario Superior Court to strike down the federal statute that blocks U.S. style drug ads on the grounds that it violates the Charter of Rights' guarantee of freedom of expression. As President of Drug Safety Canada I am party to that action—in opposition. Only two countries in the world allow open DTC advertising—the U.S. and New Zealand. New Zealand is reviewing DTC.

8   The tiny print says: "The Canadian Diabetes Association has reviewed the 'Making the Connection' program for its medical and scientific accuracy. The Canadian Diabetes Association does not

endorse the products of any pharmaceutical company." I am told by the Canadian Diabetes Association that 1. They accept non-restricted educational grants from Pfizer and other Big Pharma companies. 2. Due to complaints from their donors and members they withdrew their endorsement of the toe tag campaign after it was over, but do not participate in the current "Making the Connection" campaign. It also uses fear, featuring an angry bull, with blood filling his eye, prepared to charge a woman hanging clothes (a red flag?) on a clothes line.

9 In 2004 I found a website for the Lipid Nurse Network and called the number there. It rang at the office of one of the volunteer nurses at her job at a hospital. In other words, the "network" had no office and phone. With all due respect, it was highly unlikely they had the resources to create and sponsor millions of dollars of TV and print ads. Pfizer is still listed as a sponsor to the Canadian Diabetes Association.

10 www.eyeforpharma.com, website May 2, 2006. "Internet among most trusted sources for health information." Quoting from an Accenture Study at www.accenture.com This study showed that 60% of those that saw drug ads on TV always or sometimes trust the information.

11 *The Atlantic Journal-Constitution*, "Self diagnosis from TV drug ads can be dangerous," Bill Hendrick 01/08/07.

12 Basara, LR. "The impact of a direct-to-consumer prescription medication advertising campaign on new prescription volume." *Drug Information Journal* Vol 30(3) (pp. 715-729), 1996.

13 *Le Monde Diplomatique*—English Edition, May 2006. "Pharmaceuticals for healthy people. US: selling the worried well." by Alan Cassels and Ray Moynihan.

14 Source: www.brandweek.com "New Pharma Ad Rules Result In More Ads." May 8, 2006. Industry spinsters in the U.S. may tell you that new self-policing industry rules were introduced in January 2006 to make ads more educational and these comments are therefore outdated. But in the first two months of 2006 DTC for drugs increased by 11%, partly due to more unbranded "disease awareness ads" like the ones that Health Canada approves. Campaigns for Viagra and Levitra which appear like public service announcements urge men to call an 800 line or visit a website. This

is a move towards "relationship marketing" that target groups of patients and gets their critical data—address, phone number and email address. And some companies ignore self-regulation. Sepracor was still running Lunesta ads in 2006 despite signing on to PhRMA's ban.

15 James Lindheim, Director of Public Affairs for Burson-Marsteller, the world's largest PR company, who advise Big Pharma clients has said, "In fact the research tells us that people's perceptions of the sizes of various risks and the acceptability of those risks are based on emotional, and not rational factors ..."

Chapter 20: The Butterfly Effect

1 By Gardiner Harris and Eric Koli, June 10, 2005.
2 In 2007 Dr. Bush was made Co-Chair of the J&J Pharma Safety Council.
3 Erna Buffie & Elise Swerhone (Directors). Merit Jensen Carr & Joe MacDonald (Producers). Montreal, PQ: National Film Board of Canada and Merit Motion Pictures, 2001. *Drug Deals* won two film awards: a Platinum Remi Award in Public Health at the Film & Video Production 2004 WorldFest Houston, and Best Documentary at the 2003 Blizzard Awards.
4 *Taipei Times*, December 22, 2006. "Foundation says doctors overprescribing for kids."

Epilogue: Who Killed Vanessa?

1 Go to the Health Canada website, click MedEffect, read through the disclaimers, click "I would like to search a subset of the Canadian Adverse Reaction database" and search the database under Prepulsid. Don't forget, because it's Health Canada, search also "cisapride" which for some bizarre reason is filed separately. Remember, you are only seeing what is reported, a fraction of the real number of ADRs.
2 *Washington Post*, May 7, 2006, "Panel Faults Pfizer in '96 Clinical Trial in Nigeria Unapproved Drug Tested on Children."
3 July 21, 2007. Pharmalot website. Accessed September 3, 2007, "Nigeria Refiles Lawsuit Against Pfizer." "The Nigerian government

has refiled a $7 billion civil lawsuit against Pfizer, but this time added a more serious fraud charge to their allegations that the drug maker didn't properly obtain consent from families while testing the experimental Trovan med on their children." Reported by the Associated Press.

Afterword

1   Paxil's generic name is paroxetine hydrochloride. In the UK Paxil is named Seroxat, and in Argentina, Australia, Mexico, and South Africa they call it Aropax. Generic versions are sold under many names worldwide—at least forty. SSRI stands for selective serotonin reuptake inhibitor, and refers to the Big Pharma theory of how these drugs work. This theory has never been proven and neither has Big Pharma's pet theory about depression—that it is caused by a chemical imbalance in the brain. Remember the wording on the Prozac label: "thought to" "assumed" in Chapter 12, Games with Names? With no chemical imbalance in the brain, how would Big Pharma persuade our doctors to prescribe billions' worth of their drugs to "correct" that imbalance? You have to give the marketers credit. They have most doctors convinced.

2   *CMAJ* February 17, 2004. Dr. Jane Garland, UBC. "Facing the evidence: antidepressant treatment in children and adolescents," and *Psychopharmacology* (1996) 123:1-8 S.T. Higgins et al. "Alcohol Pretreatment Increases Preference for Cocaine over Monetary Enforcement."

3   In July 2005 GSK contraindicated Paxil with pimozide because the combination might cause sudden death—by long QT and heart arrhythmia. A fourth "Dear Doctor" letter went out in September 2005 to warn patients that Paxil was more likely to cause birth defects than other antidepressants, and in December 2005 a fifth to warn doctors again about the risks of maternal use of Paxil—heart defects in unborn children.

4   This article also showed that more than eight times as many serious psychiatric disturbances had been reported during withdrawal to Health Canada related to Paxil than any other antidepressant studied up to October 2002.

5   Eighty-eight per cent of clinical trials that showed the antidepressant

drugs didn't work weren't published in medical journals or were presented as positive findings to the FDA. Yet thirty-seven out of thirty-eight *positive* studies given to the FDA to get these drugs approved were published. The result was that doctors reading medical journals would conclude that antidepressants were *between 11% and 69% more effective than they truly are.*

6   *National Post*, March 1, 2008, Public Library of Science: Medicine Kirsch et al. Thirty-five clinical trials submitted to the FDA with data on 5,000 patients on Prozac, Effexor, and Paxil (Seroxat) showed placebo was almost as effective in improving patient's symptoms—with no risk of adverse drug reactions.

7   From SSRIstories.com: "This website focuses on the Selective Serotonin Reuptake Inhibitors (SSRIs), of which Prozac was the first. Other SSRIs are Zoloft, Paxil (Seroxat), Celexa, Sarafem (Prozac in a pink pill), Lexapro, and Luvox. Other newer antidepressants included in this list are Remeron, Anafranil and the SNRIs Effexor, Serzone and Cymbalta as well as the dopamine reuptake inhibitor antidepressant Wellbutrin (also marketed as Zyban)." SNRI stands for Serotonin-Neoprinephrine Reuptake Inhibitor, a newer type of antidepressant that also can cause severe withdrawal symptoms. Serzone was taken off the Canadian market after numerous patients on Serzone suffered liver damage.

8   A 2006 study in the *American Journal of Psychiatry* showed that artificial light therapy is just as effective in improving winter depression for seniors as antidepressants. Yet the same issue reported an eight year Ontario study that showed seniors taking Paxil, Zoloft, and Prozac were five times more likely to commit suicide during the first month of therapy than those taking other drugs.

9   I contacted Sara's father Neil. Fortunately he turned out to be a lot like me. Neil is fighting back. He is an excellent researcher and unlike me, has worked in hospitals for years maintaining and servicing medical devices and machines and is not phased by medical-speak. He is working diligently to get an inquest into the death of Sara Carlin. Neil also supports my work at Drug Safety Canada, which I founded in 2002 to promote the safe use of prescription drugs.

Acknowledgments

I sincerely thank the following people for helping me tell this story:

Gloria, Madeline, and Hart, who patiently put up with my absence and pervasive distraction while I researched and wrote this book.

Those who convinced me to write it—Jane Christmas, who also suggested the title and concept and Naomi Klein. Nancy Wood helped me make it better in many ways.

Director Erna Buffie and producer Elise Swerhone at Merit Motion Pictures who told Vanessa's story on film so beautifully in *Drug Deals* and shared the results of their thorough investigation with me.

The people at Will Barristers, especially Vanessa's champion Gary Will, who helped me in innumerable ways, Chris Morrison and Paul Cahill and cheerful the Petal Wailoo for a hundred phone calls, faxes, emails and other tasks.

Crown Attorney Brian O'Marra, who helped clarify the inquest process, and guide us all through it to its conclusion.

My good friend Canon Derwyn Shea, who helped me reconcile my faith with our loss of Vanessa and explain it to my readers.

All the people I interviewed from the beginning of my journey who were incredibly helpful, including Carol Kushner, Dr. Ray Woosley, Dr. Joel Lexchin, Dr. Neil Shear, Alan Cassels, Carol Kushner, Dr. Warren Bell, Anne Rochon Ford, Dr. Jack Utrecht, and Barbara Mintzes.

I especially thank my angels, the former insiders who bluntly told me the truth about the pharmaceutical industry, the ones I had to rename: Alex Demerse, Jane Cooper, Anna Kovacs, and Callie Hughes.

My brother, Dr. J.E.M. (Ted) Young, who is always there for advice and has always been there for our family, and my cousin Dr. David Knox, whom the people of Orangeville are so lucky to have in their community.

The public interest leaders at Public Citizen in Washington, especially Larry Sasich, Pharm. D. (now teaching at Lake Erie College of Osteopathic Medicine, School of Pharmacy along with his wife Pharmacist Sana Sukkari) and Dr. Sidney Wolfe, Larry's co-author of *Worst Pills–Best Pills*.

A group of amazingly dedicated people I met along the way in cyberspace who communicate daily to share timely information on prescription drug safety—the people on the private listserve I renamed Pharmalist. Without them I could have never come near understanding the medical-speak, pharma-speak, conflicts of interest and regulatory failures that undermine patient safety.

The public guardians in this story who put their careers on the line to keep the rest of us safe at high personal cost: Sana Sukkari and Dr. Michele Brill-Edwards.

My agent Hilary McMahon and publisher Jordan Fenn at Key Porter, who both took a chance on an unpublished writer to get this story out, and Managing Editor Jonathan Schmidt, without whose patient mentoring it wouldn't have come together.

Emma Cole, Deanna Borda, Alison Carr and Marijke Friesen who made a manuscript full of clerical errors into a readable book.

Index